HOLISTIC HERBAL
FOR MOTHER AND BABY

Also by Kitty Campion:

Holistic Woman's Herbal
0 7475 2045 3

HOLISTIC HERBAL
FOR MOTHER AND BABY

———

KITTY CAMPION

BLOOMSBURY

First published 1996 by
Bloomsbury Publishing Plc, 2 Soho Square, London W1V 6HB

Copyright © 1996 Kitty Campion

The moral right of the author has been asserted

A copy of the CIP entry for this book is available from the British Library

ISBN 0 7475 2046 1

10 9 8 7 6 5 4 3 2 1

Designed by Hugh Adams, AB3
Typeset by Hewer Text Composition Services, Edinburgh
Printed in Great Britain by Clays Ltd, St Ives plc

• DEDICATION •

To Richard Schulze, my courageous and life-enhancing teacher,
and to Victoria and Kasheen my beautiful god-daughters,
who carry the future before them.

MEDICAL DISCLAIMER

The advice given in this book is appropriate in most instances but please be aware that it is general and not specific to individuals. Any plant substance, whether taken internally or externally, may cause an allergic reaction in some people. Neither the author nor the publisher can be held responsible for claims arising from the mistaken identity of any herbs or misuse of any remedy. For serious or long-term problems a qualified practitioner should always be consulted. Pregnant women should not abandon coventional medical care for themselves or their children and should be aware that self-treatment should not be undertaken while on a prescribed course of medication until professional advice is sought. Always seek medical attention if symptoms continue. Remember that herbal medication can be very powerful and dosages should always be respected.

ACKNOWLEDGEMENTS

My heartfelt thanks to David Lawson, Agnes Meadows and Linda Harold, who have made what has been a very traumatic year joyful and positive, and who have supported me with unstinting love. Thank you to Susan Mears, the literary agent who sold a trilogy to Bloomsbury, of which this is the second volume and to Isabelle Rickard at Bloomsbury for her meticulous input with editing. Sandy Williams, my beautiful and extremely competent Personal Assistant, is the best right arm this hard working woman could wish for. Vivien and Ivan Bell extended the hospitality of their cottage in Ballywalter, Northern Ireland, while I wrote this book and opened their hearts to me. Dianne Bjarnson, who has delivered thousands of babies using only herbal wisdom and love, gave generously of her time and experience when I visited her in Utah. Richard Schulze, to whom this book is dedicated, has been my rock and firm foundation herbally and as a friend. Lastly, where would I be had Clive and Margaret Woolley not kidnapped me, adopted me and overwhelmed me with their love? I am privileged to be part of their family.

CONTENTS

PART ONE:

THE BASICS

——

CHAPTER 1:

HERBALISM FOR MOTHERS AND BABIES

Having a child is one of the most exciting and daunting events that will happen to a woman in her lifetime. Our children represent the future and all of us want the best for them. Offering your child and yourself the most you can in terms of health and well-being using natural methods which have been tried and tested throughout the centuries is one of the most important things you can do.

The prevailing attitude in the western world is that doctors deliver babies – rather than the belief that women give birth – this continues to encourage a high rate of unnatural births (including episiotomies, forceps or vacuum extractor deliveries and caesareans). Political and economic incentives tend to perpetuate the problem. The reasons for intervention are very few indeed and should be reserved for the rare occasions when Mother Nature needs a little assistance, *never* as routine procedure. Any interference with labour whether it be emotional, medical or physiological, may well muddy the process.

There has been an astonishing clash between the accelerating changes in obstetrics and in women's attitudes to childbirth throughout the 1970s and 1980s. Obstetric intervention fuelled by the use of more and more high-tech equipment has tended to overwhelm and dominate the instincts of women.

Many women are now seeking a gentler and more natural approach in a personal environment which encourages them to tap into the incredible spiritual and physical energy that pours through their bodies during labour. Prenatal care is still heavily patient-orientated and focuses on screening for myriads of problems to such a degree that the ability to diagnose defects has far outpaced the possibility of curing them, or even accurately describing how they will affect the baby. Advances in technology are not necessarily advantageous and carry with them anguish, uncertainty, inaccuracy and some hard choices. The poor foetus (let us not forget what pregnancy is all about) becomes an unborn patient and the main therapy, even supposing the diagnosis is accurate, is selective abortion.

Holistic health care is very different from this. For one thing it is incredibly empowering. It encourages, and by education, allows people to take responsibility for themselves, mind, body and spirit. The emotional changes that take place in pregnancy are almost never addressed by obstetricians yet it is possible, and indeed wholly desirable, that you help yourself through these with relaxing psychother-apeutic techniques as well as by natural therapies like yoga, massage and aromatherapy. There are many different methods you can employ to achieve optimum health and well-being at this important time including diet, exercise and herbal preparations

Lip service is often paid to diet by doctors whose training on this amounts to only a few hours throughout all their years in medical school. Taking care of yourself nutritionally before, during and after pregnancy isn't an option, it is a must. In the UK during the Second World War pregnant women were given priority in the food-rationing restrictions and even under these adverse conditions the stillbirth rate fell from 38 per 1,000 live births to 28, a drop of almost 25 per cent. If you eat well during pregnancy and put on pounds your baby is liable to be an adequate weight which greatly reduces the possibility of complications and sickness after birth. Excellent nutrition helps prevent stillbirths, low birth-weight, prematurity, infections, brain damage and retardation in babies and anaemia in mothers. Who better to advise you than a naturopath who is trained in excellent individually tailored nutrition?

Most pregnant women now know about the dangers of taking drugs during pregnancy but fewer are aware of the dangers of invasive medical checks. If problems do occur the advice as to how to solve them naturally given in Appendix I should prove invaluable and, rest assured, contra indications are listed alongside them.

Exercise is of course vital. If you do suffer from morning sickness it is tempting to do nothing and your exercise programme will often go by the board for the rest of your pregnancy. If you actively participate in some exercise before conception you can continue with it almost throughout your whole term, although you may find that you need to switch from jogging to fast walking at about six months. However, tennis, horseback riding and dancing, can continue as long as you feel comfortable doing it. If you begin to feel too heavy to exercise properly continue to do what you can. Swimming is one of the best activities for pregnant women; the water buoys the tummy up, the whole body is exercised, and it can be continued right up until birth. Several of my patients have actually been swimming on the day they went into labour. It is inspiring to note that during the Second World War when women had to take over the job of railway porters from men, those who had to take fairly heavy and strenuous exercise as a result had no problems with birthing. Their less active sisters did. Yoga is particularly recommended not simply because it includes special opening movements for the pelvis but because it leads to increased poise, self-confidence, better physical co-ordination and a wonderful sense of internal serenity and balance.

Touch is terribly important and in our strait-jacketed western cultures we seldom get enough of it. We all know those who are battered learn to batter, but have you thought about the fact that child abuse is three to nine times greater among caesarean mothers than among the general population, that it takes twelve hugs a day to optimise your immune system and that societies that give their babies the greatest amount of physical affection and touching have the lowest level of physical abuse? The touching can begin by giving yourself a massage or a do-in routine (self-administered Shiatsu); receiving a massage or experiencing shiatsu, reflexology, hellerwork, aromatherapy or manipulative therapies. But it needn't stop there.

Until the 1970s the prevailing wisdom among so-called experts was that the unborn baby could be stimulated only by touch and that its actions were reflex responses anyway. But we now know that touch develops at eight weeks, taste, hearing and smell develop at twenty weeks, response to light at twenty-six weeks and learning processes at twenty-four weeks. The Japanese have always dated age as being from the moment of conception and this is, with hindsight, more accurate than our western concept of age. Certainly it is possible to calm an uncomfortably active baby in utero with massage, aromatherapy, shiatsu and, if need be, alterations in diet, but it is also possible to communicate with your baby on all levels, spiritually, emotionally and with all your five senses. Of course it is also important after greeting your baby inside you to listen in return. Professor Peter Hepper, head of a team of researchers at the School of Psychology at Queen's University, Belfast, has proved that a 36 week old foetus who has heard a particular piece of music twice a day throughout pregnancy will react after the birth as if they had heard it before, becoming significantly more active. But babies in utero are also drawn towards light, will actively respond to massage, and react to the bitter taste of certain foods eaten by their mothers.

The best kind of holistic care is one where you can ensure a continuing relationship with a few selected caregivers only. People who you will get to know (and who will get to know you) well. A good alternative practitioner will approach you like a partner and help to build a genuine relationship with you. You should find yourself a million miles away from the doctor-knows-best attitude and you will not be allowed to abdicate your decision-making responsibilities. Good alternative therapists are neither benevolent parents or perfect caretakers. Initially, if you have been used to treating your doctor in this way (or being treated in this way), you may find this a bit scary. You may well have an exceptional doctor (and there are very many of them around) who acknowledges that although they know more about pathology, you know more about your own needs. In this case you are singularly blessed. If mutual trust governed the doctor/patient relationship the warfare that currently exists in obstetrics would largely cease. My own doctor is such an exception, and the relationship he has with the midwife who works with him at his health centre is a wonderful combination of mutual support and respect.

We are beginning to make a little progress simply because mothers and midwives throughout Europe have joined forces to press for a gentler, kinder, maternity service. Shaving of the perineum and the routine use of soapy enemas and suppositories is fairly passé. Today women are generally allowed to get up and walk around while birthing, and birth plans are often encouraged and occasionally they are even adhered to. But hospitals often have rigid hierarchies and bureaucratic rules. While I respect a woman's desire to give birth in a hospital and the innate intelligence and inner wisdom that tells her to do so, I also respect the wisdom inside any other woman which bids her to have her baby at home. The truth is very few births of healthy women require a doctor's services. It is safer to have your baby at home and by taking care of yourself holistically you should enjoy a healthy, joyful and self-empowering pregnancy.

This may sound radical, even unpalatable to some, but when you consider that 98 per cent of all births in the UK, and an even higher percentage in the United States, still take place in hospitals then I believe it needs to be said, that contrary to popular belief, hospitals may not be the safest places to give birth. For example Sheila Kitzinger, in her Home Birth Book reveals that, in Holland, where pregnant women may choose whether a doctor or a midwife attends them and where, it has emerged, that care given by a midwife at home is SAFER than care from midwives in hospitals, and safest of all is a home birth with a midwife. **This is true of even first time mothers**. Marjorie Tew, who taught statistics at the Department of Community Health at Nottingham University Medical School, tenaciously collected and courageously battled to publish these statistics and similar ones in the UK (amidst great opposition from the Government and the medical profession) and concludes, 'Complications are more likely to occur in a hospital because of, not in spite of, high tech interventions . . . the threat of a home birth is not a threat to mother and baby but a threat to the healthy survival of medical and obstetric professions.' She goes on to observe the only exception is for women at the very greatest risk, of which more in Chapter 5.

In Australia, one of the few 'civilised' countries in the world where home births are actually increasing, the perinatal mortality rate is as low as 5.9 per 1000. These figures are particularly significant because some of the women were high risk and 30.8 per cent were first-time mothers and tended to be older than average (one woman was forty-seven). Of the 8.6 per cent who moved to hospital during labour the majority did so because labour was taking a long time. The caesarean rate was 2.2 per cent (compared to the average in some parts of the United States where it is creeping up to nearly 50 per cent), episiotomies were 20.1 per cent compared to 39.9 per cent of hospitalised births.

Wherever and however you choose to have your baby all the positive information you glean from natural therapies will help you become a more effective parent.

When properly used herbs are the safest and surest medicine available. This is particularly true as far as the vulnerable and rapidly developing systems of babies and young children are concerned. However it is as well to be aware of the power of herbs both to heal and, if misused, to cause imbalance. Herbs produce no side effects whatsoever when used in the amounts required to effect a cure. Negative effects will only occur when you fall to observe the cautions that herbalists have recognised as the result of many years of experience. I stress that they should be used in the appropriate quantities for babies, toddlers, children and adults because even mild herbs can cause toxic reactions in large quantities. Herbs that are extremely concentrated such as essential oils can also be irritating in over large doses, both externally when in contact with the eyes, nose, mouth and all mucous membranes. Many of the essential oils in them are rubefacients, intended to cause a mild irritation reaction to stimulate circulation in a specific area but if they are applied to the skin in large amounts they can cause a burning irritation.

The human body from birth onwards is biologically familiar and metabolically compatible with whole plant foods and medicines. The body is capable of using such plant constituents as foods and building materials or it will actively excrete them. It is this predictable act of excretion by various eliminative organs of the body that gives human kind the medicinal uses of the actions of individual plants. The tunnel vision of the isolated active ingredient of a plant used in allopathic medicine just does not do what the subtle complexity of the plant does. Herbalism is therefore much safer for young growing bodies than the harsh actions of allopathic medicine. Provided the herbs used are of good quality, harvested correctly, prepared, compounded and properly prescribed, the actions of each herb are 90 per cent predictable. An experienced herbalist knows what whole herbs singularly or in a complex formulation can do and what they cannot do. The 10 per cent variability stems primarily from the person's lifestyle and how this lifestyle stacks up against the action of a herb. Children have the added advantage of not having polluted or corrupted their systems too much. In my experience babies and children react very pleasingly, quickly and positively to herbal medicine.

In this book I hope to show you how to take a responsible and extremely empowering approach to the natural process of pregnancy and birth which, after all, is a normal physiological process, not an illness. The constructive information in this book is intended to help parents create healthy happy babies and by healthy I mean the well-being of the whole child, mental, social, emotional, physical and spiritual.

The habits that children acquire from birth on wards and the skills they learn, particularly in their first five years, will shape their bodies and may well influence the kind of diseases to which they are susceptible. Parents are the lynch pin of their child's health and growth because they are the baby's models. They shape the overall nature of the baby's environment which is, in turn, inseparable from the parent's own growth and fulfilment.

CHAPTER 2:

THE HERBAL PHARMACY

―――

I always think of women during pregnancy, birthing, lactation and the subsequent business of bringing up babies and young toddlers as being at both their most vulnerable and their most potent, and for this reason I am particularly careful when administering herbs at this stage of a woman's life and during infancy. For example, I will not use tinctures during the first trimester or give them to babies simply because even the smallest amount of alcohol is disturbing to the body. I prefer to give herbs in tea form and will occasionally use them as poultices or in powdered form in capsules. During birthing, however, I will nearly always rely on tinctures because they enter the bloodstream so rapidly.

• PROPORTIONS OF HERBS FOR TEA MAKING •

The standard proportions are 1 tsp of dried herbs or 2 tbsp of fresh herbs to one cup of water or 1 oz (30 g) of dried herb to 1 pint (600 ml) of water. The proportion of fresh herbs can be increased to 3 oz (90 g) to the same amount of water. Remember water will only extract the water soluble principle of the herbs and if you are using fresh herbs they should be gently crushed between the fingers or with a stainless steel knife or bruised in a pestle and mortar. Crushing them in this way brakes down the cellulose of the plant. Dried herbs may need to be further pounded or chopped in a pestle and mortar. Water-based preparations decompose rapidly so they should be made freshly every few days and any excess should be stored in the refrigerator in a glass jar or china basin covered with muslin or linen. This will help the preparation to breathe.

• HOW TO DETERMINE DOSAGE •

If the problem is chronic (marked by long duration or frequent recurrence) estimate 3 to 4 cups of tea daily. If it is acute (characterized by a sudden onset, sharp rise and short course) take a quarter of a cup of tea once or twice an hour until the symptoms subside while awake. If using a tincture for a chronic problem estimate 15 drops three times a day and note that a tincture is usually put into some other carrier base such as water or juice before drinking rather than put straight on the tongue, simply because it tastes so strong. The exception to this is if you have mouth ulcers or a sore throat in which case specific herbs can be very helpful sprayed directly on to inflamed membranes. For an acute problem take 10 to 15 drops of tincture every half hour until symptoms subside. Powdered encapsulated herbs are normally taken with meals for a chronic problem, two size 00 capsules three times daily. If the problem is acute one or two capsules every hour until the symptoms subside. If it is uncomfortable to take this number of capsules over several hours ensure that you are swallowing them with a fruit smoothy or some pureed fruit. This will provide added ballast to the stomach and make them easier to digest.

When giving herbal remedies to babies and children the dosage should be decreased proportionately. As a general rule the dose should follow the body weight so that a 40 lb (18 kg) child will get no more than half the dose of an 80 lb (36 kg) child. All doses recommended in this book are adult doses calculated to suit a body weight of about 150 lb (68 kg). Therefore women weighing less than 150 lbs (68 kg) should begin with a lower dose. Proportionately and logically a child weighing 75 lbs (34 kg) would take half the dose of an adult weighing 150 lbs (68 kg). Therefore if a 150 lb (68 kg) woman is asked to take 15 drops three times a day, a 75 lb (34 kg) child would take 5 drops three times a day. Herbs for babies are best administered either by bathing them in the appropriate herbs, applying them externally in fomentations or poultices or through breast milk. In my experience breast-fed babies will take herbs in infusion or decoction form in a dropper but they generally don't take to this kind of dosage terribly kindly.

• METHODS OF TAKING HERBS •

Herbs can be smelled, swallowed, injected into any bodily orifice (such as washing the eyes out or using an enema), gargled or applied to the skin, either by rubbing them on in ointment, cream or oil form, or by using them in water as part of a hydrotherapy routine. I have often found water treatments the best medicine of all for babies and toddlers, and although fasting is not normally recommended during pregnancy it is often one of the surest ways of getting a pregnant woman through a crisis (providing it is supervised by a professional medical herbalist and done for a maximum of between one and three days). I have, for example, had a woman fast in her seventh month of pregnancy for three days while doing a gall bladder flush simply because she had no choice. Her gall stones were so painful and she wanted to avoid an operation. The flush was extremely successful and the baby was none the worse for it. However, I stress again that fasting during pregnancy should only be used in emergencies and guided by an experienced naturopath or professional medical herbalist. In these instances I would always choose an organic fruit juice fast. Some tribes will fast on water for 24 to 76 hours in order to induce birth believing it gives them strength to go through the birthing process.

INFUSIONS

These are made with the more fragile parts of herbs including flowers, leaves and stamens. The normal method is to weigh out the herbs appropriately (see page 8–9) and cover with freshly boiled filtered water, stirring the preparation (but not with anything aluminium) and covering the container tightly to leave it to steep for a minimum of 20 minutes. The preparation can then be strained through muslin, nylon, or a stainless steel or silver tea strainer. It will be accepted more easily into the body if it is drunk warm rather than icy cold or very hot. Any excess can easily be warmed to the correct temperature.

DECOCTION

Very tough leaves or seeds, roots, barks and berries need a more rigorous process to ensure the active constituents are released into the water. Begin by crushing them with a pestle and mortar or a coffee grinder before use. The only exceptions are burdock root and cinnamon sticks which simply need steeping in freshly boiled water but not boiling water, and golden seal and valarian roots, both of which are very high in volatile oils and are best infused rather than decocted. You will notice that decoctions will generally stay fresher for longer than infusions. Having prepared your herbs cover them with cold water in a non aluminium or copper saucepan with a tightly fitting lid and bring the mixture to the boil very gently continuing to simmer for 15 to 20 minutes until the water is reduced by half. Strain as above and use as required.

If a formulation requires both the tough and tender parts of herbs mixed together simply prepare it by first decocting the tough bits and then turn the heat source off and add the herbs to be infused, allowing the mixture to steep for a further 20 minutes before straining.

All herbal teas can be sweetened with honey, maple syrup or black strap molasses or diluted with fruit juices of your choice to make them more palatable if necessary, but women who are already aware that they may be hypoglycaemic or suffer from gestational diabetes should avoid sweeteners. Teas intended to nourish or detoxify the liver should be taken in their original form because tasting the bitterness is part of the process of healing.

All herbal teas made in this way will normally last for two or three days if stored in a cool place, but if you notice an odd taste or bubbles forming on the surface of the tea throw it away as it will no longer be usable.

TINCTURES

Alcohol is a better solvent than water and has the added advantage of acting as a preservative but I stress again that I feel that herbal tinctures should not be used during pregnancy, except nearing the time of birth and during the birthing process itself, nor should they be administered to babies and toddlers. Besides being taken internally, tinctures can also be rubbed into the skin directly or applied on poultices previously dampened with water. Some very high-quality herbal tinctures are readily available in health food stores (see Resources Directory) and any professional medical herbalist you choose to consult will have an even wider range.

The medium (or menstruum) used for tincture making can be alcohol (usually good quality brandy, gin or vodka). Never use alcohol in the form of surgical, spirit or methanol as these are extremely poisonous. Wine is not acceptable for tincture making because its alcohol content is too low, nor are you advised to buy even the various delicious herbal wines available while pregnant. When making tinctures from alcohol buy the best alcohol you are able to afford, preferably anything which is 80 to 100 proof. Because alcoholic tinctures are so rapidly assimilated by the body their affects are quickly felt.

GLYCERIN TINCTURES

Their disadvantage is that they don't dissolve resins or oily plant constituents although they do preserve the parts of a herb you would normally use for infusions extremely well. Buy Glycerin which is 100 per cent vegetable origin as glycerin made from animal fat is hard to digest and is not intended for human consumption. It is usually used in cosmetics. When using glycerin use 2 parts to 1 part of water and proceed as for alcoholic tinctures.

VINEGAR TINCTURES

I particularly like these for people who are very sensitive to alcohol and especially for children. Not only is vinegar non toxic but it helps to regulate the acid-alkaline balance of the body and has the added bonus of acting as a tonic for the digestive system. Use 100 per cent organic apple-cider vinegar if you can get it, or if you can't, wine vinegars are the next best thing. Malt, distilled or balsamic vinegars are absolutely not acceptable. Apple-cider vinegar will draw out the valuable alkaloids, vitamins and minerals from plants but cannot draw out important plant acids.

All tinctures once made should be stored in dark glass bottles and kept in a cool dry place, tightly stoppered. If you do this they will last for three or four years.

Fill a glass or stainless steel vessel three quarters full with fresh chopped or pulverised herbs (you can use dried, but fresh are preferable). Cover with the appropriate menstruum adding an additional 2 to 3 inches (5 to 7.5 cm) more to the liquid so the herbs are totally and fairly generously immersed. This allows them room to swell as they soak up the liquid and if they start to peep above the liquid just add more menstruum. If using vinegar, warm the vinegar first slightly. Cover with a tight fitting lid. Shake vigorously and keep the container somewhere warm; an airing cupboard is ideal. Try and remember to shake the whole mixture well daily or twice daily if you have the time and strain after fourteen days.

Tinctures should be started with a new moon and strained with a full moon, fourteen days later. The power of the waxing moon helps to extract the medicinal properties more effectively. (There are diaries that chart the course of the moon which can be obtained from local stationer shops.) At the end of the appropriate length of maturation time strain the herbs through cheesecloth using the cloth to wring out every drop of tincture. The herbs can be used for composting. Rebottle the tincture into smaller bottles remembering to cap tightly and label. Keep them away from light and heat.

If you are using an alcoholic tincture and want to avoid the alcohol contents simply add it to boiling water removing the water from the heat source and let it sit uncovered for five minutes before drinking.

HERBAL OILS

These are readily obtainable from health food shops and your local professional medical herbalist. Garlic oil, borage and evening primrose oil and wheatgerm oil can all be bought in capsules. I make a deep heat oil which is superb for mastitis, lower back pain and sports injuries. But its preparation is very difficult so I would not advise the amateur herbalist to consider it.

OINTMENTS AND CREAMS

While you can make these yourself reliable ointments and creams are readily obtainable from health food shops or your local medical herbalist. They are particularly effective for dry and cracked skin and need to be applied generously and rubbed in thoroughly. Creams, because they are lighter and more easily absorbed, are better for treating sore, chapped skin or protecting and moisturising healthy skin.

PESSARIES

T-tree pessaries are readily available from health food stores and are excellent for treating thrush, vaginally or anally. They should be used every night, one being inserted before going to bed and renewed nightly for a week to do their work well (see Resources Directory). It is fine to use pessaries during pregnancy.

SYRUPS

These are the most delicious of all the herbal preparations, particularly as far as children are concerned, and they act as great tonics, soothing sore throats and helping with digestive problems. However, they require a lot of prolonged heating and large quantities of a sweet carrier base and this disturbs the medicinal action of most herbs, so except for cough and cold syrups and when making syrup of ipecacuana they are not my method of choice.

Method

To a strained decoction add one quarter of its weight in liquid honey, preferably organic, then stir it over a low heat until the honey is dissolved. You may need to skim off the rising scum occasionally. Decant into labelled glass bottles. Syrups will last for several weeks and sometimes even months if stored in a refrigerator.

POWDERED HERBS

Because the whole herb is used in its powered form, not an extract, these are usually the most potent and effective form of herbal medicine. However, their disadvantage is that when powdered leaves and herbs are exposed to oxygen and moisture their important active constituents are rapidly broken down and they have a maximum shelf life of a year only. Also, powdering fails to break down the cell walls which are difficult for our digestive systems to process, so they are not advised for those with poor digestions. Powdered herbs can usually be bought ready prepared and packed in capsules (very few of which are now made out of animal products). But in some instances, it is essential to taste the herb (as when taking bitter herbs for the liver). If you need to taste the herbs put them in a little warm water and stir and drink immediately. You can buy herbs already finely powdered from the suppliers listed in the Resources Directory. These are available in various sizes – for an adult the correct size is usually 00. To fill the capsules first spread the herbs onto a shallow dish, then ensuring your hands are completely dry, separate a capsule in two and fill both ends with the powdered herbs. Then stick the capsule back together. Store capsules in glass jars away from heat and moisture because moisture will ruin them.

Some people find swallowing capsules difficult and if this is the case place the capsule on your tongue with some water and then bend forward from the waist and swallow a little more water. The capsule should slide back gently and easily into the throat. (For capsule suppliers see Resources Directory.)

POULTICES

These are particularly useful for applying nutriment directly through the skin via the lymph and blood circulation to the tissues and organs beneath. They are also a good way of softening and dispersing material that has become hardened such as breast lumps. You will need:

1. Herbs. Fresh herbs need to be liquidised in a little water; dried ones should be macerated in a little hot water; and powdered can stay simply as they are.
2. Slippery elm powder, arrowroot or cornflower as a carrier base.
3. Apple cider vinegar, preferably organic.
4. White, fine, pure cotton. A very large man's handkerchief usually does beautifully, depending on the area to be treated. Gauze is also suitable.

5. Two large plates and a large saucepan of boiling water.
6. Plastic sheeting (such as a piece of bin bag or those plastic bags that come from the dry cleaners) stretchy cotton bandages and safety pins.

Estimate enough herbs to cover the area to be treated to a depth of quarter of an inch (6 mm). Mix these with about a tablespoon of the a carrier base in enough apple cider vinegar to form a thick paste. Spread the piece of cotton on to a plate and put this over a saucepan of boiling water. Scrape the herbal mixture on to half the cotton, keeping it from the edge to stop it squelching out when you use it. Fold the other half of the cotton over the top, then fold the damp edges together and press out any excessive moisture. Cover the whole with the other plate until the poultice is really hot. Remove and apply as hot as bearable to the affected area, but obviously don't burn yourself. Cover with plastic; secure with bandages and safety pins or, if the area is very large, a thin towel. Leave on all night, particularly if there is material such as bolls which need drawing out. If the poultice has to be applied somewhere on the trunk wear a tight cotton T-shirt which will help to hold it firmly in place.

Next morning peel the poultice off and warm it up using the plate method. Meanwhile clean the area by bathing it in a warm decoction of diluted apple cider vinegar, half and half with purified water. Reapply the poultice but this time use the other side against the skin. Repeat each evening with a completely fresh poultice (using it again in the morning) until the area is healed.

ENEMAS

I often get negative feedback about enemas from those female patients who have experienced an enema just before childbirth (usually not voluntarily) administered amidst fear and discomfort and often using soapy water which induces violent and painful peristalsis (as well as destroying all the benign flora from the colon). Let me reassure you. An enema if correctly administered is easy to carry out and reasonably comfortable. What you need to do is to allow yourself plenty of time and privacy and lay out everything in advance because the more relaxed you are the easier you will find the whole process. I have used enemas on pregnant women to relieve morning sickness both in the first and the last trimester, to induce labour and in cases of chronic constipation, although in this instance I would prefer to administer a colonic irrigation. Colonic irrigation uses 15 gallons (68 litres) of purified water held at a specific temperature to wash out the colon. Administered gently and a little at a time, it is thirty-two times more powerful than an enema. If a woman has gone through a series of colonics preconceptually or had some while pregnant in my experience they normally encourage a strong but very speedy labour. A professional colonic irrigation therapist will know when not to administer a colonic to a pregnant woman. (For a list of colonic therapists see Resources Directory.)

Let me dispel some myths about enemas. They do not make a mess. Your anal sphincter is perfectly capable of holding liquid in the colon until you decide to release it. Initially it is common for the stimulation of the enema fluid in the bowel to make you want to rush straight to the toilet and release it but you will acquire self control with practice.

Taking an enema is really quite logical. You wouldn't dream of unblocking a drain from the top end of the waste pipe and in the same way a blocked colon needs to be relieved from the bottom end first. If you have a fever an enema is the surest and quickest way to relieve the bowel of toxic waste. If you are so weak you cannot eat, an enema can supply nourishing superfoods to the digestive tract and this is particularly useful in cases of severe morning sickness. Heavily pregnant women when taking enemas towards the end of their term should lie on their left-hand side with their knees bent up. It is best when you are this heavily pregnant to get a friend to help to administer an enema. Lobelia enemas just before going into labour are particularly helpful.

You will need:

1. Three and a half pints (2 litres) of a herbal decoction or infusion made with filtered water. Cool enemas are used for cleansing and warm ones for treating nervousness and spasms.
2. An enema kit (see Resources Directory).
3. Olive oil, Vaseline, or KY jelly.
4. A large bath towel or a piece of plastic sheeting.

How to take an Enema

1. Fill up the enema bag with your chosen infusion or decoction at the right temperature and hang it from a hook in the bathroom at shoulder height.
2. Lubricate the tip well with Vaseline, olive oil or KY jelly.
3. Lie down on your right side with your knees tucked up to your chest and gently push the lubricated tip of the enema tube into the rectum. Don't worry it won't slip in too far because it is joined to the kit with a tap which acts as a barrier.
4. Release the tap and allow the liquid to flow slowly into the rectum. If the liquid encounters a block of impacted faeces you will feel marked internal pressure so turn off the tap, and massage the area in an anti-clockwise direction.
5. When you are half-way through the mixture (and you will know this by keeping your eye on your bag suspended from your hook),
carefully roll over onto your back with your knees bent and place the soles of your feet flat on the towel or plastic sheet beneath you. When the enema pack is emptied of its contents turn off the tap and remove the nozzle tip.
6. Carefully stand up and wrap yourself in a bath towel then go and lie down on your bed with your bottom raised on some pillows. If you are nervous about spilling any of the enema mixture onto your bed cover the bed first with a plastic sheet.

7. Retain the enema for 20 minutes if you can. Get up and release whilst sitting on the toilet.
8. When you are ready to wash out the enema kit using natural soap and hot water, dry it with a towel and allow the tube to drain by hanging it over a hook. It can then be put back into its surrounding carrier-bag and if it is made of rubber, sprinkle with a little corn starch to stop it sticking together before packing it away.
9. The golden rule is never share your enema kit with another person. It is entirely personal to you.

> *Enemas should never be relied upon to replace your usual bowel movements, nor should they be abused by over use. It would not be acceptable to take an enema every-day to remedy constipation, for example. I would consider this over-use. Enemas are excellent to take waste out of the system in an emergency, such as a high fever, headache, etc.*

> *Pregnant women should never douche and should not douche for at least a week after delivery. Women who experience pain while douching should stop at once. Persistent vaginal infections should be reported to a doctor or a professional medical herbalist and can be appropriately treated with pessaries and creams used externally as well as sitz baths and herbs administered orally.*

• THE HERBAL MEDICINE CABINET •

A good herbal medicine cabinet and a portable herbal medicine first-aid bag is a boon to every home. All of the preparations mentioned can be bought from your local health food shop or by consulting your local medical herbalists should you not have the time to indulge in creating one and its contents are clearly discussed in Chapter 9. In the Resources Directory there is further advice about particularly excellent sources of commercially made herbal preparations. Remember your first and foremost rule should always be to consider the quality of the herbs that you are using. Whenever possible try to buy organic or wild crafted herbs which are far more potent than non-organic ones. Your choice here will help encourage the steady growth of an industry striving to provide excellent quality. In addition you will be discouraging the widespread use of chemicals and helping to support small companies.

Labelling is very important. If making herbal remedies yourself do list all the ingredients on a label from the most to the least important one. Include instructions and whether it is for internal and external use. Put the date you finally completed the product on the label, too, so you know how long it can be stored safely. If a label falls off, for whatever reason, unless you are a very experienced herbalist I would advise you throw the preparation away rather than take any risks.

When making formulations yourself do not use either aluminium or copper. Aluminium is extremely poisonous and copper will destroy the vitamin C content of certain herbs.

• HOW SAFE ARE HERBS DURING PREGNANCY? •

Most herbs are remarkably safe to use during pregnancy. Not only do herbs provide a brilliant source of concentrated nutrition but because they have a natural composition their high vitamin/mineral content is readily assimilated. My own experience shows with many of the labours of my patients that they are extremely helpful in easing pain and assisting throughout, and after birthing they readily help to restore the vitality and strength of the mother and iron out any problems the baby may be experiencing.

I have noticed a lot of herbals carry huge lists of herbs that shouldn't be used in pregnancy, which can often be very offputting to the amateur. My golden rule is: if in doubt always consult a professional medical herbalist. The following herbs are best avoided because, for one reason or another, they are toxic during pregnancy.

ALOE

While aloe juice taken internally can be useful to help with mild constipation and to heal internal ulceration the dried sap of either curacao, Barbados or Cape aloes should not be taken by pregnant women as they are rich in emodin and will cause contractions of the uterus thereby risking miscarriage. Aloe vera gel can be beneficial when massaged into the skin to help minimise stretch marks, and is a wonderful soother for burns, rashes, psoriasis, insect bites and itching. It should not be taken internally.

ANGELICA

Useful for menstrual irregularity. It does, however, cause uterine contractions and is therefore only used by herbal midwifes during childbirth when labour is delayed or prolonged. It is a wonderful herb for helping to expel the placenta after childbirth.

AUTUMN CROCUS

This should be administered by a trained medical herbalist as large doses can produce violent nausea, diarrhoea and stomach irritation.

BARBERRY

Only to be used under the supervision of a trained medical herbalist as, although an excellent urinary antiseptic and diuretic, it also oxytoxic and may stimulate the uterus inappropriately.

BETH ROOT

The beth root, commonly known as birth root, was successfully used by the red Indians to ease pain during childbirth as it helps to stimulate contractions and get the birthing process moving properly. But for this reason it should not be used during pregnancy.

CELERY SEEDS

Made as a decoction these can act as a uterine stimulant and so should be avoided during pregnancy.

COLTSFOOT

Coltsfoot contains pyrrolizidine alkaloids and should be strictly avoided during pregnancy.

COTTON ROOT

Freshly picked this is high in oxytoxins and at one time was used to induce abortions. It is also believed that for men with low sperm counts it acts as a male contraceptive, reducing the levels of testosterone, although as yet this hasn't been satisfactorily proved. Avoid it.

FALSE UNICORN

Again this contains substances which mimic a hormone that can help to bring on labour so should not be used during the course of pregnancy except under the professional guidance of a medical herbalist (see page 191).

GOLDEN SEAL

This should not be taken by diabetics because it lowers blood sugar levels. It should also be treated with caution by hypoglycemics because after more than three consecutive months of usage a previously unaffected person may begin to exhibit the symptoms of diabetes. Taken long-term it will stop the absorption and digestion of B vitamins in the digestive tract. It should not be employed for prolonged use during pregnancy because it contracts the uterus but it can be superb as an aid during childbirth.

JUNIPER

Juniper berries are wonderful for clearing up a brief attack of cystitis if chewed fresh or dried but they should never be used for prolonged treatment during pregnancy.

LIMETREE FLOWERS

While limetree flowers are not contra-indicated in pregnancy always ensure your supplies are fresh as old fermenting leaves and flowers can cause hallucinations.

BLACK COHOSH

Again, like Angelica, black cohosh is not for use until the last few weeks of pregnancy. It is a superb uterine tonic but has a stimulating affect on the uterus. It is often combined with blue cohosh (see below) because of its unique properties which enable it to stimulate contractions while at the same time relaxing tension and stress that can collect in uterine muscles.

BLUE COHOSH

Blue cohosh is a strong uterine stimulant like black cohosh and should not be used until the last few weeks of pregnancy, but it is particularly beneficial if labour is prolonged.

MUGWORT

Because Mugwort relieves menstrual obstruction and has an affinity for the womb it is not to be used during pregnancy or while lactating.

MALE FERN

Dioscorides, an ancient Greek herbalist, was aware of its power to induce abortion and infertility and although it is seldom used today, it must not be taken during pregnancy.

MARIGOLD

While generally an excellent and very useful herb, Marigold should only be used externally during pregnancy because it promotes contractions and delivery of the placenta.

MOTHERWORT

Though helpful during the last few weeks of pregnancy, Motherwort promotes menstruation and therefore should not be used during the proceeding months following conception.

NUTMEG

Although perfectly acceptable in small quantities in cooking, in large quantities the poisonous alkaloid, strychnine, can result in fatalities and it should not be used during pregnancy because it can induce abortion.

PENNY ROYAL

The leaves of this herb are perfectly safe to take during pregnancy but the essential oil can cause abortion and should be avoided.

POKE ROOT

While, as a professional medical herbalist, I have used this successfully as an emergency measure during pregnancy, you should be aware that it contains substances that distort cell structure so it should always be taken under the professional guidance of a medical herbalist during pregnancy.

SAGE

Sage oil contains toxic keytone as part of its essential oil complex and if consumed regularly over some months may produce womb spasms and the possibility of an abortion.

SASSAFRAS OIL

This oil is carcinogenic and to be avoided.

SHEPHERDS' PURSE

Not to be taken during pregnancy because it stimulates the uterus but is unbeatable for stemming uterine haemorrhages that occur afterwards.

TANSY

This should not be used during pregnancy as it stimulates the uterus.

TOBACCO

Avoid it at all costs before, during and after pregnancy, especially if breast feeding and try not to breathe in other people's tobacco smoke (see pages 21, 70, 78–9, 82, 184).

YARROW

This causes uterine contractions and should not be used during the first trimester. Generally it is a very safe non-toxic herb and superb for colds and fevers. It also acts as an excellent haemostatic and is often used in combination with Shepherds' purse to arrest haemorrhaging during childbirth.

• STORING HERBS •

Anything made with alcohol, vinegar or glycerine will keep for at least a year if stored in an opaque, well-stoppered glass bottle. But herbal formulae, no matter how effectively dried or preserved, all grow less effective with age. In my own pharmacy the herbal powders, pessaries and boluses are made up weekly but then I see a fair number of patients. You will probably not be able to turn your stock around so quickly, so remember to throw away any dried herbs (except roots, berries and barks) once they have passed their first birthday.

Syrups will keep indefinitely as honey is an excellent preservative. Even so I would advise you to store them in the fridge. Essential oils will keep indefinitely in opaque glass bottles but air gaps should be eliminated as they are used, by transferring them to smaller and smaller jars. Poultices and fomentations should always be freshly made. Cotton bandages and sheets should be well boiled after use, dried, and stored in plastic bags. All herbal preparations should be stored in glass containers – never plastic ones, which absorb other smells and disintegrate under the influence of essential oils.

You will soon know when herbal preparations have gone off. They smell odd, fizz or turn ominous colours, in which case treat your compost heap to them. My guiding dictum is 'If in doubt throw it out'. To save yourself the expense of doing this, buy only a few ounces of the herbs you need at a time unless your family is enjoying lots of certain teas you have grown. It is better to share with a friend than to be landed with stale stocks. I know communities where one person volunteers to grow a few herbs and another some different ones, and these get shared around as needed, which seems sensible.

CHAPTER 3:

DIET – THE BEDROCK OF GOOD HEALTH

Never doubt it. Information is power and the quality of any decisions you make about your health before, during and after pregnancy, depend on the quality of your information. The information I am about to give you about your diet during pregnancy may appear at first sight to be unconventional but it is scientifically ratified and has been physically proven over many years by thousands and thousands of healthy pregnancies and birth.

• THE FAR-REACHING EFFECTS OF MATERNAL NUTRITION •

A good diet just before conception and during pregnancy greatly increases the possibility of producing a healthy baby, so taking special care of yourself nutritionally both before you conceive and throughout your pregnancy and lactation isn't merely optional, **it is absolutely vital**. Excellent nutrition helps every single aspect of conception, pregnancy and birth. It lowers the risks of everything from low birth-weight, prematurity and eclampsia to caesarean sections, and is proven to result in fewer still births, better brain development, fewer learning disabilities and healthier babies. My entire work is founded on the bedrock of nutrition and during the course of my training I came to appreciate that the basis of all good health is excellent diet. So the advice I am about to offer you may sound radical but its wisdom has been proved by naturopaths all over the world since 500 BC. It is not intended to stress you or make you feel inadequate or guilty. Simply regard it as the best possible advice you could get on nutrition just before and during pregnancy and decide how much of it, if any, you want to make your criteria.

Everything we eat or drink must be assimilated or eliminated by the body and both processes need energy. Our main energy drain is digestion. If we ingest more toxins or waste than the body can handle the body becomes enervated. If the nerve energy is depleted the brain is forced to assign priorities. The process of elimination and detoxification is slowed or checked so that internal toxins and metabolic waste start to build up. It can build up to a level where the integrity of the body is in question. Then the body begins a purging process through its eliminative channels.

We create auto-intoxification by ingesting more toxins, food or waste, than the body can eliminate at speed. So what causes disease is toxemia or enervation. It is possible to put in more poisons than can be eliminated and they build up biochemical additions which the body cannot use. Naturopaths therefore see disease as a cure. An uncomfortable cure certainly, but a philosophically sound and time-proven cure nevertheless.

To eat excellently so that you and your baby are truly nourished you need to:

- combine foods effectively
- eat fruit properly
- break your fast (literally breakfast) to your maximum advantage
- avoid eating when stressed
- eat comfortable amounts of foods
- avoid drinking water with meals
- eat organic whole foods whenever possible
- never eat just before bed
- eat according to your cicadian rhythms (of which more later)
- eliminate fats, animal flesh, dairy and acid forming foods from the diet, all of which naturopaths consider to be poisonous addictions

Now most people reading this list may reluctantly go along with the first nine principles, even if they have only the haziest notion of what they may entail, but they baulk at the tenth. The main question I get asked is 'why?', closely followed by 'what does this leave me to eat instead?'. So let's deal with the biggest issue first, and I will deal with it entirely on health grounds, although, goodness knows, there are tremendous issues of environment, ecology and compassion which are equally valid.

• FATS AND OILS •

Saturated fats, which only come from animal flesh, and coconut and palm kernel oil are the major cause of heart disease which is responsible for one out of every two deaths throughout the entire Western world. Saturated fats cause our red blood cells to stick together so that they can't flow through the capillaries properly and oxygen does not reach them. The cells begin to weaken, die, mutate or clot. If they clot oxygen can't reach them at all and the result is a heart attack. If the blockage is going towards the brain the result is a stroke.

Fats and oils contain over twice the calories of proteins and carbohydrates. Nine calories per gramme compared to only four calories per gramme of carbohydrates or proteins. A diet high in saturated fat will elevate the triglyceride level in your blood increasing the risk of atherosclerosis (when the arteries start to clot up as the result of excessive cholesterol build up). This has been recorded in babies as young as nine months. Indeed an epidemiologic study performed by the Department of

Medicine, Louisiana State, University Medical Center, showed yellow fatty streaks and cholesterol accumulation, both significant signs of early atherosclerotic clogging of the arteries in *most* children under the age of five. In a study carried out in Derby by Osborne (1963), a local pathologist, he reported on over two thousand deaths in young people by coronary thrombosis and also noted that out of sixteen cot deaths the only baby who had normal coronary arteries was the one who was breast-fed.

So during the course of your pregnancy and while lactating you should aim to cut right down on saturated fats.

WHICH OILS ARE THE HEALTHIEST?

Choosing the best vegetable oils instead is as simple as looking at their extraction process. Always choose one which is closest to nature and has the least processing or alterations. Most commercial oils that are clear, light and tasteless have gone through over two hundred physical and toxic chemical processes in their production. Often extremely high heat, well over 212°F (100°C) is used in many phases of the extraction along with extremely toxic chemicals. These chemicals, one of which is caustic soda (as used in chemicals to unblock drains) are used to extract, refine, bleach, de-gum and even deodorise oil. At some point in the process oil is heated to over 500°F (260°C) for up to an hour. This oil is still sold as cold pressed because external heat was not used during the initial pressing stage. Amazing deception!

CHEWING THE FAT

There are many types of fats but they all fit into three basic categories, saturated, mono-unsaturated and poly-unsaturated. Vegetable oils contain all three of these types of fat, but are classified in the group where the highest percentage of their fat occurs.

MONO-UNSATURATED OILS

While all oils contain percentages of saturated, unsaturated and mono-saturated fats, your oils of choice should be those with the highest percentage of mono-unsaturated fats. These are olive oil 82 per cent, peanut 60 per cent, canola 58 per cent and sesame 46 per cent. The problem with canola oil, currently the darling of the health-food industry and often used to replace palm and coconut oils, is that it is marketed for good cardio-vascular health. But canola oil contains urucic acid which has been found to cause fatty degeneration of the heart, kidney, adrenals and thyroid. In contrast olive oil has actually been proven to raise levels of HDLs, high density lipo proteins, and it has been the oil of choice of natural medicine for thousands of years. Studies have shown that in countries where olive oil consumption is highest, like Italy, Spain and Greece, death rates due to coronary artery blockage and cancer are reduced, besides which, olive oil was the first oil used by ancient Greek and Roman cultures because it could be extracted using the simplest pressing methods. Choose the darkest green olive oil you can find. The darker the colour the less it has been processed. Once open store it in a cool place away from light.

OMEGA-3 FATTY ACIDS

Omega-3 fatty acids, otherwise known as EPAs or N-3 fatty acids, have been proven to prevent blood clots and coronary artery spasm and prevent the development of coronary artery blockage. What is less commonly known is that the famous Eskimos who eat them have among the highest rate of haemorrhagic stroke in the world, that is paralysis or death caused by a haemorrhage in the brain and that Omega-3 fatty acids actually *raise* cholesterol levels.

The most well-known source of Omega-3 fatty acid is, of course, fish oil, but these oils generally come from fish which are contaminated with pesticides, heavy metals, chlorinated hydrocarbons and, in some parts of the world, sewage and other waste. Fish oils rot easily due to oxidation. The poisons in them are particularly concentrated in livers and the liver is the organ that processes and tries to neutralise chemical toxins. In diabetics fish oils actually cause insulin resistance and raise blood glucose levels. Remember too the warning on page 00, and if you are pregnant, diabetic and like fish, stick to white fish only, plaice, cod, halibut, sole, etc.

The good news is that Omega-3 fatty acids are naturally present in wholegrains, beans, walnuts, pumpkin seeds, flax seeds, seaweeds, soya beans. Obviously, wholegrains, walnuts, pumpkin seeds and soya beans are very easily obtainable, but overall flax seed contains 58 per cent Omega-3 fatty acid; double the quantity available from nuts, grains and seed sources combined. It can be easily digested during pregnancy by grinding the seeds up in a coffee grinder and stirring the resulting coarsely powdered mix into soups, cereals and soya yogurt. An added bonus is that flax seed is wonderful for healing and cleansing the colon, of which more on page 99. So choose only *vegetarian* sources of Omega-3 fatty acids.

SAFE FRYING

The problem with deep frying is that oil kept at 215°C (419°F) for 15 minutes or more has been shown to unfailingly produce atherosclerosis in experimental animals and in food shops that specialise in deep frying operations, the same batch of oil is often kept at a high temperature for days at a time. Some of the substances that result from this are toxic, the effects of many have yet to be discovered, but you can safely bet none of them will improve your health.

A safe alternative is to add the vegetables to the pan *before* adding the oil to protect it from overheating and oxidation, or to add a little filtered water to the pan *before* adding the oil. This way the resulting steam protects the oil from air and the temperature is kept down to 100°C (212°F). Either way the food tastes less burnt and more flavoursome. Cooking like this requires your presence and attention, but it does pay dividends as far as your health is concerned.

Let's get this straight. We *need* oils in our diet. It is one of the vital food groups necessary for our continuing health. During pregnancy oil is needed as an energy source for constructing and maintaining vital organs of the growing baby such as the brain, heart and kidneys. The only two fats absolutely essential for mother and baby are linoleic and linolenic acid and these are richly abundant in nuts, vegetable and nut oils as well as nut butters, pulses, wholegrains and avocados. Oils derived from cottonseed or rape seed oil (commonly called canola oil) should be avoided. They contain harmful contaminants including gossypol and ururic acid which can damage internal organs. Coconut and palm kernel oils (which are often present in commercially baked goods) should be avoided as they are saturated fats. The oil contained in oily fish has been associated with decreased blood clotting ability, a potentially dangerous problem during labour. Women who consume large amounts of oily fish have a greater risk of the pregnancy being prolonged past term. This potentially allows the baby to become abnormally large, and frequently causes birth complications.

Oil deficiency may manifest itself as dry skin, dandruff, seborrhea, lustreless hair. More silently it is needed for the proper working of the bile ducts and in the production of adrenal and other hormones. But fats basically make you fat, and excessive weight gain is as dangerous during pregnancy as being severely underweight. Every unnecessary pound increases the risk of diabetes and the delivery of overly large babies who may suffer from birth trauma or, in the medical profession's opinion, require delivery by caesarean section.

So the message is that the total number of calories in your diet which come from oily substances should not exceed 25 per cent daily and this is *not* a problem as there is so much naturally present in the foods already cited. You have to go to incredible measures to deprive your body of the fat it needs. If you take it in concentrated forms (liquid oils and nuts and nut butters) try and make sure it is entirely unsaturated and nonhydrogenated.

MARGARINE VERSUS BUTTER

Margarine is made by a process of hydrogenation in which hydrogen gas is bubbled through polyunsaturated oil in the presence of a metallic catalyst, usually nickel or cadmium, until it solidifies. It can be made rock solid if enough hydrogen is used, the very process of hydrogenation turns it into a saturated fat. So much for the cunning advertising which implies it will actually *prevent* heart disease! In fact margarine *causes* a steep rise in cholesterol, and deaths from heart disease and cancer are highest among people who eat margarine.

Think, for a moment, about what margarine actually is. When examined under a microscope it has the same molecular structure as plastic. It will not melt when you squeeze it or rub it in your hands. No microbes will attack it nor will it grow mould in the usual way, which means it is an entirely *dead product*. Now, logically, what will your bloodstream do with such an unnatural substance? There are a few totally nonhydrogenated fats on the market which are solidified with lecithin. **Read the labels**! Any label that says 'high in polyunsaturates' plays down the fact that hydrogenation is in itself a saturation process. Look for the words non, not or unhydrogenated. The fats made in this way are fine in moderation.

● THE REASONS FOR CUTTING DOWN ON MEAT ●

This is not a moral or an environmental issue, although I could make it so if I chose to and that, in my opinion, certainly has some validity. But it is a protein issue as far as pregnant women are concerned. The whole subject of protein is simply groaning with myths. Protein *does not* give you energy. It is the *last* thing our bodies use for energy. The first thing that the body burns is sugar, the second thing is carbohydrates. Protein is only used as a last resort. Excess protein creates surplus nitrogen in the body and nitrogen creates fatigue.

Protein *lowers* endurance which is why marathon runners load up on carbohydrates before a race for energy and endurance. Protein does *not* give you strong bones. Vegans have been shown to have much stronger bones than flesh eaters. Osteoporosis has now been proven to be the result, not of calcium deficiency, but protein excess. Calcium loss occurs for hours after a flesh meal because the kidneys must lose calcium as they cleanse the blood of excess protein waste, a condition called protein-induced hypercalciuria. There is now impeccable evidence proving that excessive protein from flesh foods leads to kidney hypertrophy, inflammation and a much higher incidence of kidney stones.

DANGERS OF EXCESSIVE PROTEIN

World health statistics show that osteoporosis is most common in exactly those countries where dairy and flesh are consumed in the largest quantities – the USA, Finland, Sweden and the UK.

The Eskimo diet, laden as it is with fish, fish bones and meat, produces the osteoporosis champions of the world. Physically active vegans very rarely suffer from osteoporosis.

Vegans live longer than flesh eaters who also suffer from higher rates of cancer of the breast, prostate, pancreas and colon and both of these facts have been known for a long time.

HOW MUCH IS ENOUGH?

We grow faster during infancy on mother's breast milk than at any other time in our lives yet breast milk is only about 2–4 per cent protein at birth; and it reduces to 1.2–1.6 per cent within six months. Even as adults we need very little protein. Various experts ranging from the American Journal of Clinical Nutrition to the World Health Organisation estimate a daily intake of protein somewhere between 2.5 to 8 per cent. Interestingly mothers milk falls pretty much half-way between these two ranges which just shows what a perfectly balanced food it is.

WHERE DO I GET MY PROTEIN FROM?

There is protein available in practically everything. Wheat for example is 17 per cent protein. Oatmeal 15 per cent. Cabbage 22 per cent. Pumpkin 15 per cent. Potato 11 per cent. Arnold Schwarzenegger recommends 1 g for every 9 kg (2 lbs) of body weight and if you ate nothing but cabbage all day you would *still* be getting four times his suggested requirement (and probably very bored with a mono-diet to boot!). So the idea that plant protein is somehow incomplete is a myth.

Nature is incapable of creating a food without using every amino acid required by humans. There is a famous vegan community in Tennessee called The Farm where 800 babies were safely and healthily delivered. The pregnancies, birthing and subsequent particularly exuberant and trouble free health of all these mothers and babies has been well documented. So your protein intake throughout pregnancy should be from non-flesh or dairy sources if at all possible and will be amply met without much worry on your part. During the last trimester it would be wise to take 10 per cent of your daily intake as protein. The reason? Pre-eclampsia has been attributed to insufficient protein intake. However vegan mothers are much less prone to pre-eclampsia anyway, but a small increase of protein at this stage is a prudent and cast-iron strategy.

Sprouted seeds are a particularly wonderful nutritive protein. All seeds, grains and pulses can be sprouted and should at the very least be soaked overnight before their use in any meal preparation. This soaking or sprouting process greatly increases the content of usable protein and raises the active vitamin content by several hundred per cent. It also helps to make beans and seeds more digestible as the enzymes in them are activated by the sprouting process, changing the starches to simple sugars. Pregnant women should resist the temptation to eat more than 2 oz (60 g) of any sprouted food daily, because there are plant alkaloids, particularly in alfalfa sprouts, that may adversely affect the mother and baby if eaten in excess.

WHAT ELSE IS IN MEAT?

The US Department of Agriculture reports that 37 per cent of chickens carry salmonella, a figure that has been pretty constant for the last ten years. Four per cent of all beef and 12 per cent of all pork is contaminated but because chickens are coprophagous (they eat each other and their own droppings) salmonella is a common inhabitant of their intestines and rarely bothers them. But when the chickens are killed their entrails are often nicked allowing salmonella to spread. The spraying of the carcasses with chlorinated water reduces the bacterial count, but not much, and the current method of screening relies mainly on visual signs of infection but as we all know you cannot see bacteria with the naked eye.

Animal flesh contains measurable and still active quantities of female hormones (oestrogens and stilbesterol) fed to the animal to increase weight, fat content or egg production. So when you drink your milky coffee or eat your steak and eggs you may be washing traces of these potent sex hormones through your baby in utero.

Meat, fish and dairy products all commonly contain hydrocarbon chemicals as well as PCBs and PBBs (polybrominated biphenyls). These are all toxic residues from industrial pollution or the agricultural spraying of pesticides which gather in the flesh and milk of animals fed sprayed feed grains and given polluted drinking water. So what they consume you eventually eat yourself, and, as they accumulate in breast milk, your baby gets to eat it twice over, once in the womb and once out.

How you cook your meat is also important. A study supported by the Dutch and US governments concluded that the most important mutagens (substances which cause cancer) in diet are the product of overheating meat. Fried meat results in a really big increase in mutagens both in the blood and urine and the Japanese National Cancer Centre has long been advising its public not to overheat meat. So if you eat meat it should be boiled, braised or steamed.

I appreciate there will be some of you who enjoy eating meat and want to do so throughout your pregnancy so if you like meat cut down a little:

1. Eat a small piece only once per day.
2. Choose leaner cuts and cut the fat off.
3. Eat meat you are certain has been naturally raised without the use of any kind of chemicals whatsoever. However it is essential to understand that while meats labelled 'natural' or 'organic' may well be better than the typical factory farm commercial products they still include the concentrated toxins from all the foods the animal ate. These accumulate in animal fatty tissue in much greater concentrations than are found in fruits and vegetables.
4. Boil, braise or steam it, and if using it in soups or stews prepare the dish, chill and skim off the fat before reheating.
5. Keep the implements you use for preparing meat separately and wash and dry them separately. Chop meat on a surface that can be scoured and store all uncooked meat in the fridge well away from other foods.
6. Always combine it properly with other foods. Remember meat does not mix with starch or fruit.

MEAT SUBSTITUTES

1. Tofu which is made from soya milk solidified with nigari (the residual concentrate from sea water when sea salt is extracted from it). It is solid and chewy for those missing the texture of meat and readily available in packets from supermarkets, health-food stores and oriental grocers. Simply store it in the fridge (some tofu is packed in water, in which case spill out the water, cover with fresh water and store in a closed container, changing the water daily until it is all used up).

   Tofu is very bland in flavour so will readily acquire the taste of any sauce or seasoning with which it is mixed. Unlike other proteins it is alkaline not acid and because it doesn't have any crude soya bean fibre it will combine properly with starches.

It is entirely cholesterol free, high in amino acids and contains more calcium than milk. It is also abundant in B-complex vitamins, vitamin E, choline, iron, magnesium, phosphorus, potassium and sodium.

It can be blended with fruit to make yogurt and unlike natural yogurt is not sharp in flavour. Silken tofu which imitates cream is available in pouring packets and makes an excellent substitute for cream or custard or as part of a fruit fool, ice cream or mousse (though I have to say it tastes nothing like cream). Tofu can be mashed with tahini or tamari for a savoury salad dressing, mixed with turmeric to make omelettes, blended into gravies, used as a binder in cake batters and casseroles, mashed and seasoned as part of a sandwich spread, sliced and sautéed as cutlets and, of course, diced, marinated and stir fried in vegetables sautés.

2. In the USA there are some amazing meat substitutes made from wheat gluten (the protein part of the wheat) which are so authentic I'd defy you to differentiate them from the real thing. They even look like the real thing (chicken breast, frankfurters, bacon, etc.) and some of them are slowly creeping into Europe. It is possible to eat in certain Chinese restaurants where wheat-gluten meat is used exclusively and this is advertised on the menu.

3. Shitake mushrooms, fresh or dried and soaked, are not only brilliant for boosting the immune system (the Japanese use them as an anti-cancer medicine) but have a meaty texture and complement rice or pasta beautifully. Tossed in a wok with a little oil they are satisfyingly crispy (for those missing pork crackling and roasted chicken skin).

4. TVP and other dried soya-based substitutes exactly mimic mincemeat. Again remember to reconstitute them by soaking and season well to add flavour. They do not combine with starch being rich in soya fibre.

5. Finally always remember vegetables and grains are so infinitely versatile you really never need feel deprived eating out or in. Try Mexican bean burritos, Chinese stir-fries, Japanese vegetable tempuras, Italian marinara and primavera sauces, luscious breads and pastas, grilled vegetables in a carvery (you'll need to speak to the chef in advance), Middle Eastern pitta breads with all sorts of delicious fillings, Spanish guacamoles, iced soups, salads. The only countries I've ever had trouble eating out in (and I travel a lot) are France and Germany who still lean heavily on meat and fish – but even they are learning and I've eaten sensational and imaginatively prepared and presented vegetable platters at bistros in France, and satisfyingly thick vegetable and bean soups in Germany with some tasty breads.

• DIAL M FOR MILK, THE MISGUIDED LEGACY OF DAIRY PRODUCTS •

Think about this. Cows don't drink milk, calves do. So why do you? We are the only mammals on earth that go on drinking the milk of another species throughout our adult lives. Cows' milk is naturally designed to turn a 45 lb (20 kg) calf into a 3000 lb (1360 kg) cow in a year. At that speed an 8 lb (3.5 kg) baby would weigh 89 lb (40 kg) at two years old. So the powerful growth hormones in milk are certainly not needed for humans.

The protein in cows' milk is mostly casein which forms hard, indigestible curds in a baby's stomach. The protein in mother's milk is mainly lactalbumin which babies can easily digest. This is exactly as it should be. Cows are big, fast-growing and genetically very distant from humans, and nature, in her perfect wisdom, has designed the milk of each animal species precisely to meet those nutritional needs of the young of that species. Baby zebras don't suckle adult giraffes!

Yet milk is the most political food in the Western world. We are brainwashed into believing milk is wholesome and good for us when the truth is precisely the opposite.

MILK IS INDIGESTIBLE

- Milk and all milk products tend to neutralise the stomach's hydrochloric acid which forces your stomach to work harder and harder to digest food.
- The enzymes needed to break down and digest milk are renin and lactose and these have virtually disappeared by the time we have reached three. It is estimated 20 per cent of Caucasian children and 80 per cent of black children and adults are severely lactose intolerant and experience abdominal cramps, diarrhoea and dehydration due to drinking cows' milk.
- An even greater percentage find that the casein coagulating in the stomach puts a tremendous burden on the body to expel it and a huge amount of energy is spent dealing with this, so habitual dairy intake can often make you very tired.

MILK AND ALLERGIES

Cows' milk allergy is not a recent discovery. Hippocrates noted that milk could cause gastric upset and urticaria; Galen recorded allergy to goats' milk and since the revolution of the dairy industry and the introduction of infant formulas based on cows' milk, allergy has become much more prevalent (though it is still seldom recognised by the medical profession). Nor is goats' milk any better for those intolerant to cows' milk.

The bovine protein in dairy products, once swallowed, is smeared on throat membranes, tonsils, adenoids and other gateways into the immune system. Some of this protein can cross the surface membranes, and when the protein from another animal is introduced into the human immune system an allergic response is triggered in many parts of the body.

This is why dairy products are so notoriously mucus forming. It is simply the natural reaction to an assault by a foreign protein. The resulting mucus flow creates chronic runny noses, persistent sore throats, bronchitis, recurrent ear infections, hoarseness, sinus congestion and headaches. More insidiously excessive mucus is generated in the intestines, hardens and forms a coating which is relatively impermeable to nutrients. This means poor absorption and leads to chronic fatigue.

Other body membranes such as those lining the lungs and joints, can react too and with the swelling and inflammation comes asthma and rheumatoid arthritis. It has long been well known that patients with asthma and rheumatoid arthritis, including my own, improve dramatically when taken off diary products.

In my experience low-grade allergic problems like eczema and psoriasis often prove to be reactions to various animal proteins. I've even observed breast-fed babies react with various allergies if the mother herself is on dairy products. In a study carried out by Gerard over a twenty-five year period, seventy-three breast-fed babies were found to react to foods eaten by their mothers, mainly cow's milk and eggs, and once the mothers stopped eating these the symptoms of the babies were relieved whatever bodily system was involved.

OTHER POISONOUS SUBSTANCES IN MILK

Some milk also contains antibiotics and 20 per cent of milk-producing cows in the USA are infected with leukemia viruses, which are not only resistant to killing by pasteurisation but have had to be withdrawn from supermarket supplies in the past. Now here's an interesting statistic. The highest rates of leukemia are found in children aged three to thirteen and the occupational group with the highest rate of leukemia is dairy farmers.

Other dairy products

Cream, which is both seductive and versatile, can be frozen and sold as ice-cream, congealed with mould and turned into cheese, aerated and churned into butter, mixed with sugar and cocoa and sold as chocolate and fermented with bacteria into yogurt and sour cream. All these cream-based products will clog your arteries, contribute to weight gain and encourage elevated hormone levels that may foster cancerous growths.

Do I hear any cries for the low-fat virtues of cottage cheese? Sorry. Apart from being burdened with all the numerous disadvantages of milk it is generally thickened and set with calcium sulphate, known to you and I as Plaster of Paris.

Cheese is a particularly concentrated food. It takes five quarts (5.5 litres) of milk to make 1 lb (454 g) of cheese. Its protein is responsible for many migraines. Yellow cheeses are soaked in chemical dyes. If you must, eat white cheeses and eat them with vegetables only. That way you have at least a fighting chance of passing them through your digestive system without taxing it too much.

If you wish to eat ice-cream at least eat the real thing in total isolation, for the same reason. Most ice-cream is a travesty of this. Cream is seldom used. It is replaced by cooked tallow, suet and lard, that is offal and scraps from abbatoirs which have the fat boiled out of them. Enough additives are added to support a chemical factory but for some odd reason manufacturers are not required, by law, to list additives.

Yogurt, lauded as a health food, is just as bad. If you're eating it for all that healthy lacto bacillus you'd need to eat 16 fl oz (450 ml) in one sitting to get even a fraction of an ounce intact and unattacked by digestive juices to reach your lower colon where the lacto bacillus in it is most needed. It has all the disadvantages of any dairy product and more as commercial yogurt has various forms of gelatine and vegetable gums added for thickness. All these denature yogurt, whether it is gelatine, agar-agar or guar gum. Supermarket shelves are increasingly packed with fruited yogurts with sugar, artificial flavours and colouring. A common use with fruited yogurt is the phrase 'no sugar added', which disguises the fact that the fruit preserves originally purchased by the yogurt manufacturer to flavour the yogurt *already* have the sugar and corn syrup added by the fruit-preserve manufacturer.

The list of non-yogurt ingredients found lurking in frozen yogurt would not embarrass a chemical factory and includes sugar, corn syrup, sodium citrate, polysorbate 80, vegetable gum, gelatine, carboxymethyl cellulose, mono-and di-glycerides, artificial flavours and artificial colouring. Commercial frozen yogurt, especially the thickest and creamiest, may not have any live yogurt culture added to it whatsoever.

For those of you worried about missing out on replenishing the colon with lacto bacillus garlic does this more than adequately (see pages 57–8) and has many other additional bonuses besides. Our digestive tracts, if healthy, house 3–5 lbs (1350 to 2270 g) of a rich variety and complex balance of 400 different types of bacteria and outside factors such as diet, antibiotics, high noise levels and stress can upset this delicate balance. Strains of acidophilus and bifidus need to be from human sources if they are to be effective in the gut and they have to be high enough to actually make a difference.

Neither is the case as far as the much touted bio yogurts are concerned. Dr Anita Ramping, a medically qualified microbiologist and Head of the Public Health Laboratories in West Dorset, says, 'I doubt whether cultures would colonise the gut and stay there.' Of the nine different bio yogurts recently tested by Consumer Checkout only three contained satisfactory levels of lactobacillus acidophilus – AB live natural yogurt, Natural bio yogurt and BA Live low-fat set yogurt. So again, if you do eat yogurt, please don't be misled by the cleverly worded labels which bend an imprecisely worded law.

INFANT SOYA MILK

Phytoestrogens which are found at high levels in soya products are naturally occurring hormone mimickers which some researchers claim could have detrimental effects on a baby's development. It seems that a baby fed exclusively on soya milk would consume as much as 20 mg of phytoestrogens a day and on a weight for weight basis this is three to five times higher than the amount of phytoestrogens from soya that has been found to disrupt the menstrual cycles of women in other studies. A New Zealand Health Ministry internal briefing paper, obtained under the Official Information Act, lists possible health effects of toxicants in soya as 'growth depression, immunosuppression, abnormal responses to hormone stimulation and cancer', but does conclude that it would be difficult to establish actual harm to consumers and that much more research is needed. My feeling is that it is safer to wean young babies on to carrot juice, homemade nut milks using organic nuts and, if pushed, goats milk. I see no harm in feeding young children diluted soya milk in moderation but certainly more research needs to be done in this area as the jury is still out on this.

WHEY

This is the by-product of cheese production. It looks like pus and tastes appalling and, I can put it no other way, it stinks. Only 10 per cent of the milk needed to make cheese actually ends up as cheese. The rest is separated out as unlovely whey and the cheese industry have to get rid of it somehow. But the problem is whey is so toxic it cannot be poured into sewers (it is two hundred times stronger a pollutant than residential sewage) and very few ordinary sewage works are capable of treating it. If it is dumped in streams it leaches out all the oxygen and kills the fish. Put into landfills it may seep into our water supplies. So it is put into baked goods, ice-cream, luncheon meats, imitation chocolate, soup mixes and beverages. Ovaltine, for example, contains more whey than any other ingredient except for sugar. So again, read your labels! If you like hot milky drinks try carob powder or syrup mixed into heated soya milk. Pureed dates or prunes taste remarkably chocolatey as a substitute in baking.

SUBSTITUTES FOR DAIRY PRODUCTS

1. Anything made of milk, butter, cream, cheese, ice-cream and yogurt is adequately and deliciously substituted by soya products which you can find in good health-food stores. The only item that still needs some work is soya cheese. They tend to do it better in the USA and Germany. Nor does it cook or heat terribly successfully. But every other soya product does.
2. Rice milk is also available in some health-food stores and combines well with cereals.
3. A Champion juicer, or equivalent powerful juicer makes sensational ice-cream (simply press frozen fruit through it substituting the blank for the screen). A liquidiser with very sharp blades works almost as well, but the end result inevitably is a little more lumpy. Banana ice-cream is delicious, and peach, raspberry, pineapple, mang and kiwi fruit taste good too. Alternatively make a smoothy (recipe below) and freeze to a slush, then liquidise, refreeze in trays, cups or individual ice-lolly moulds.

Fruit Smoothy

300 g (10 oz) frozen juice
1 frozen banana, peeled
1 cup frozen berries

● Liquidise and drink. Added ice will turn it into a slush.

4. Tofu (see pages 29–30, 37, 129) can be used as a substitute for yogurt and cream. It can be transformed into sour cream by using lemon juice.
5. Nut milks taste amazing and as children grow bigger (although nut milks are very good for young babies too) and need something cool, light and easy to digest, they're ideal in all departments. The secret is a really good liquidiser with sharp blades and **very** cold water.

Nut Milks

Half a cup of any shredded nut or seed
1 cup ice-cold water

● Blend at high speed until smooth (about 90 seconds). Add sweetener to taste (optional) e.g. maple syrup, concentrated apple juice, etc.

● You can mix your nuts and seeds, use half nut butter and half nuts, whatever you like.

Banana Milk

3 sliced ripe bananas
2 cups ice-cold water
One and a half tablespoons tahini
1 tablespoon maple syrup, barley malt or other sweetener (optional)
half teaspoon natural vanilla

● Blend well (about 30 seconds). This is superbly rich in easily assimilated calcium.

● FISH ●

Unhappily fish now tend to live in contaminated waters so they are tainted with measurable doses of cancer- and mutation-producing substances, including hydrocarbon pesticides and radioactivity from nuclear wastes, both of which produce severe cell mutations.

Heavy metals like lead and mercury which can produce kidney damage in mothers and cause blindness and mental retardation in foetuses are becoming a frequent modern malady and pesticides have been found in mothers milk. I've already mentioned problems with fish oil (see page 25) but there is the equally worrying one of parasites. According to ABCs *Prime Time Live* in the USA broadcast on the 2 March 1994 two thirds of all fresh fish tested was technically rotten with bacteria and parasites. (This was in spite of the fact that it looked, smelled and tasted fresh.) Another two thirds tested positive for toxic levels of PCBs, and a quarter had toxic levels of mercury.

Pollution is becoming a dangerous problem causing cancer, liver disease, skin disease and various-viral infections in fish. While you may think you are not likely to eat fish like this the simple truth is you wouldn't know.

In 1978 the Thames Water Authority discovered hermaphrodite fish in the river Lee which supplies drinking water to London. The effect on rats of drinking sewage was studied for eight years – before the results were deemed 'unsuitable for publication'.

The Ministry of Agriculture, Fisheries and Food carried out similar research in 1990. They found that rainbow trout and carp mutate when exposed to low levels of sewage and oestrogen hormones from contraceptive pills. But they didn't tell anyone about this for two years and then the results were buried in the obscure Foundation for Water Research Journal. New research is funded by private industry and therefore covered by commercial confidentiality clauses.

So if you enjoy your fish and want to continue eating it in pregnancy try and get it from the deepest part of the cleanest oceans like the Pacific and Antarctic. Buy it fresh, not frozen, don't deep-fry it, and ask your fishmonger where it came from.

● EGGS ●

Most among us will remember a British politician losing her job because she spoke the truth about the salmonella epidemic in eggs. Eggs are very high in fat and cholesterol and virtually fibreless. Weight for weight they contain eight times the cholesterol of beef. Eggs are also super glue inside and outside the body and, if anything, bond even stronger than the paste made out of casein to stick up wallpaper. The walls of Venice were built out of eggs and mud more than five hundred years ago and they are still standing!

Eggs are laid by hens that are fed arsenic to kill parasites and stimulate production. Eggs are rich in sulphur which strains the kidneys and the liver (and the nose if you have ever smelt a bad one!). The vast majority of eggs are tortured into existence so if you must, at least do hens the courtesy of buying free range. They are also such a concentrated protein that they should **never** be mixed with other proteins and, of course, never with starch (see page 28).

EGG REPLACEMENTS

1. When baking, two tablespoons of liquid equals one egg. So use water or whatever liquid seems appropriate for the recipe. I've found thin soya cream an excellent substitute in baking.
2. Soya mayonnaise bound with lecithin, not eggs.
3. Tofu is a good egg substitute. Try the following tofu omelette.

Tofu Omelette

240 g (8 oz) cake of tofu, washed and drained if necessary
3 tablespoons nutritional yeast
1 tablespoon tamari
2 tablespoons olive oil
quarter of a teaspoon of turmeric

- Mash the tofu then stir in the other ingredients. Tip into a frying pan and spread out evenly with a slicer. Brown on one side and then the other. This will serve two.

- To make this into a Spanish omelette add 1 onion, finely diced, 2 cloves of crushed garlic and 1 red pepper, finely diced, sauté all three ingredients in a little extra oil first.

What does all this dietary advice amount to? I believe that if you want to eat the healthiest diet in the world during pregnancy, become a vegan. In my clinical experience with 12,000 patients over the last fifteen years, women who are vegans throughout their pregnancies have easier labours and deliveries, are generally healthier and their babies are a reasonable size but not too large. Their skin is leaner and more resilient so they seem to get fewer stretch marks, they suffer less morning sickness and their craving, if anything, tends towards the healthy not the peculiar. Look too at the compelling argument for remaining a vegan whilst breast-feeding on page 00.

I do acknowledge that vegetarian eating isn't for everybody. It seems many people have adapted better than others to having a lot of meat in their diets and such people may feel wonderful when they first switch to a vegetarian diet but can then find that the feeling of super energy vanishes and somehow they never feel totally well again.

The initial good effects are similar to those from a fast. A meat-free diet has far less toxins and requires less energy to digest but some people who come from generations of meat eaters both crave and to some degree need meat and in this instance should have small quantities. We are, of course, all individuals and slavishly following another person's diet can lead to disaster. There is no one ideal diet that suits every single person on the planet.

Being a vegan or near vegan confers a lot of health benefits and morally has plenty to commend it. But please be sensible. If you are used to substantial amount of animal-based foods every day don't switch to vegan eating overnight. Substitute vegan meals for meat meals gradually, and give yourself time to adjust. If you feel you need meat don't feel guilty about it but for your sake and the sake of the animals you are eating try to find a meat, poultry or fish supplier who treats all living creatures with the respect that they deserve.

If the arguments I have presented for becoming a vegan, at least during the course of your pregnancy and while lactating, do not convince you, then move towards eating a wholesome organic diet, moderate your intake of meat, eggs, fish and dairy products and observe the following advice.

• FOOD COMBINING •

Ivan Pavlov in his ground-breaking book *The Work of the Digestive Glands* (1902) conclusively proved that every kind of food provides a specific type of gastric and intestinal secretion. Because the presence of three concentrated foods (protein, carbohydrate and fruit, for example) calls for antagonistic chemical processes at the same time, it is a physical and chemical impossibility for the digestive glands to function properly because they are governed by definite laws. So if you want to truly assimilate your food and make full use of it, it needs to be ingested in specific and optimum combinations.

If we don't do this the partially digested food can produce harmful toxins which place strains on a body trying to off-load the poison. Besides which the one process that uses the most energy in our body is digestion. It takes up more energy than running, swimming or cycling. So if we treat our digestive processes kindly our organs will not be prematurely exhausted.

Different kinds of food need different types of digestive juices and not all of these juices are compatible. Starchy foods (like rice, barley, wheat and potatoes) need an alkaline environment for digestion. Proteins (nuts, soya beans) need an acid solution for digestion.

If you mix a starchy food and a protein together (dates and nuts, eggs and chips, beans on toast) both acid and alkaline digestive solutions are simultaneously produced. They neutralise each other and digestion grinds to a halt or, at best, is impaired. The starches ferment causing a souring of the stomach and gas, and if you keep this up you may end up with a stomach ulcer.

If you wake up exhausted even after seven or eight hours of solid sleep every night you may well be hypoglycaemic (see pages 102–3) but you may simply feel that way because your long-suffering digestion has been doing the graveyard shift trying to digest the incompatible mess sloshing around inside you. This can go on for fourteen hours. Ever burped the taste of the previous nights meal? Properly combined foods digest in only three or four hours.

SOLUTION

- Try to eat only one concentrated food in a meal. That is any food that is not water-rich. Water-rich foods embrace **all** fruit and vegetables except squashes, pumpkin, potatoes and legumes which count as concentrated foods because they are more dense and solid.
- Do not eat protein and starch mixed together.
- Do not mix fruit and starch. **All** fruit should be eaten in isolation and on an empty stomach. This is because it is so high in water, and as such it is incredibly cleansing and leaves behind no toxic residue. It is supremely easy to digest. In fact it doesn't digest in the stomach it is predigested and sweeps through the stomach in twenty minutes releasing its supercharged nutrients into the small intestine and into the bloodstream. Fruit juice acts even more rapidly as an energy boost.

All this applies to fresh fruit and freshly squeezed juices. Baked, canned, stewed or dried fruit does not have the same nutrient value, nor does cooked juice or juice with added chemicals.

Allow twenty to thirty minutes to pass before putting anything else into your stomach and let three to four hours elapse if you have previously eaten anything other than fresh fruit.

● CYCLICAL EATING ●

As the Chinese have long known our bodily rhythms are circadian. The eliminative organs, particularly the liver, are working flat out at the complex processes of detoxification from 4 a.m. until midday. Why then would you want to interrupt this vital process with an improperly combined hearty traditional breakfast? The sensible thing to do is to have only fresh fruit and fresh juices and herbal teas till midday. If you suffer from morning-sickness or hypoglycaemia you may like to add the superfoods to your juice (see pages 49, 53–60, 76, 129) for additional insurance and choose ginger tea with honey and lemon (see page 87).

From midday until approximately 8 p.m. is the most suitable time for taking food on board and if you've ever eaten a very late meal you'll remember how uncomfortable this makes you feel.

The time your body really gets to digest food is 8 p.m. to 4 a.m. providing it is properly combined. If it isn't it will struggle on a lot longer than that. If you are hungry in the night eat any amount of fresh fruit and juices but *nothing else.*

Initially all of this may seem mind-bogglingly complicated but please try it and see, even if you decide not to be vegan during your pregnancy. Just observe the simple food-combining rules and physical ones and I **guarantee** your energy will rocket. Just as importantly in the last trimester (when some of my pregnant patients have felt they resembled beached whales and felt as torpid) meticulous food-combining pays handsome dividends both in terms of ease of digestion and consequent comfort and energy.

• WATER WITH MEALS •

Do not drink water with your meals. It dilutes and therefore weakens the digestive process. Carbonated water may taste more exciting than plain water but carbon dioxide is a waste gas which your lungs are constantly breathing out so why cram it into your digestive tract? It will cause wind, discomfort and burping.

Since water makes up 80 per cent of your body your diet should consist of lots of water-rich foods and pure water. Water-rich foods are fresh fruits and vegetables and their freshly squeezed juices as well as fresh sprouts. Being pregnant is a very watery state. In pregnancy you need additional blood for you and your baby as well as an additional three to six quarts (3.5 to 7 litres) of amniotic fluid in the uterus. Other sources of water include soya milk, nut milks, herbal teas, coffee substitutes and, of course, pure water itself. Water-rich foods are designed to simultaneously cleanse and nurture your body. The cleaner your body the more effectively it will work for you.

QUALITY OF WATER

Clean water, it seems, is no longer our God-given right, yet next to air clean water is the second most precious commodity for our good health. Since a pregnant woman's blood volume increases by more than 40 per cent over the course of her pregnancy a vital part of her prenatal care, perhaps the most important part, is ensuring that the blood volume is adequate. So it is actually healthy for a woman to retain more water than usual during pregnancy – a condition known as physiologic oedema. Any synthetic drug such as diuretics given to reduce this water retention and the swelling which accompanies it can actually inhibit the vital increase in blood volume. In addition, taking diuretics can disturb the body's system of salt, water and potassium metabolism as well as placing added stress on the kidneys. When blood volume is low (hypovolaemia) the placenta cannot function properly, leading to growth retardation of the foetus, birth defects and poor implantation of the placenta which, in turn, can lead to the placenta breaking away from the uterine wall (abruptio placenta) before the baby is born. But I must point out that although these disorders are serious they are extremely rare, so please don't worry about them too much.

So I stress again, plenty of fresh clean water is essential during pregnancy. Yet millions of people in Britain are currently drinking water contaminated with levels of toxic chemicals that are frequently far in excess of international standards. So far, over 350 different man-made chemicals have been detected in British tap water.

As yet we know far too little about the affects of such industrial chemicals on our drinking water except that they are acknowledged carcinogens. There is little doubt that nitrates can cause methemoglobinaemia in bottle-fed babies, a condition where the baby in effect suffocates because the blood cannot contain sufficient supplies of oxygen. The last recorded case in the UK was in 1972. Yet almost twice as much nitrate fertiliser is applied per hectare of farmed land as was used fifteen years ago and its insidious leaching into the water supply takes years, so we are only just reaping the legacy of nitrates applied in the early 1980s.

There have also been cases of sub-clinical illness caused by oxygen starvation in the blood of very small babies. In *Britain's Poisoned Water* (Penguin, 1989), Frances and Phil Craig cite a study conducted in the USSR which looked at a group of older children who drank water with a nitrate level only half of the EC permitted limit. Not only did they have slower than normal reflexes, but they were all found to have raised methemoglobin levels in their blood hindering the development of their central nervous systems.

In high nitrate areas like Yorkshire and East Anglia bottling plants purifying water for babies and pregnant women have had to be established.

• LEAD •

Lead is a neuro toxin and can damage the brain and nervous system causing anaemia and effect the muscles. High levels of lead in water have been demonstrated to depress the intelligence of children. In 1987 the Government Medical Research Council concluded from a study commissioned in Edinburgh that most city children probably had lead levels in their bodies high enough to impede their intellectual growth and that 'there is no evidence of a safe level'. Lead absorbed from water running through lead pipes was frequently the main source of the poison.

Studies by the Greater Glasgow Health Board in 1980 have shown that mothers with a higher than average level of lead in their bloodstream suffered more still-births and that surviving babies tended to be born very small. Lead poisoning from tap water is still widespread in schools and hospitals. A senior water scientist reported in 1983 finding lead levels of 5,000 micrograms per litre in the children's ward of a hospital.

Other types of piping – iron, plastic, copper, lead, zinc and cement – containing asbestos – are also known to cause problems. The effects are heightened when the water is soft because soft water is more acidic than hard water and more likely to leak out dangerous trace elements like lead or cadmium.

Our water contains other medical wastes, including natural and synthetic steroids, such as oral contraceptives and certain anti-cancer drugs. Governmental bodies concluded that the ingestion of hormones offered no risk, but recommended periodical analysis in case there is a build up of synthetic hormones in re-used water sources.

• FLUORIDE •

About 10 per cent of the population in the UK and 50 per cent in the USA drink fluoridated water which has been associated with cancer, genetic disorders, brittle bones and mottled teeth. The problem is most of us overconsume fluoride from natural sources such as food and drink as well as artificial ones like insecticides, anaesthetics and preservatives. The difficulty is that only half of all ingested fluoride can be excreted by the average healthy adult, and children, diabetics and those with debilitated kidneys may retain as much as two thirds of their ingested fluoride. This build-up in the body is associated with bone-related cancer, liver/bile cancer, oral lesions, abnormal cell changes and metaplasias (replacement of one tissue type with another). The link between fluoride and brittle bones has long been established but even very low levels of fluoride inhibit the ability of lucocytes (infection-fighting white blood cells) to migrate, which means fluoride depresses the immune system. Infant formulae made up with fluoridated water can contain up to one hundred times the amount of fluoride obtained from mother's milk.

Unfortunately there are, as yet, no filters on the market able to remove fluoride so if you live in a fluoridated area drink bottled spring water.

The following symptoms may indicate a fluoride overload.

● Chronic fatigue not relieved by extra sleep or rest
● Headaches
● Dryness of throat and excessive water consumption
● Frequent need to urinate
● Aches and stiffness in muscles or bones
● Muscular weakness and spasms
● Gastro-intestinal disturbances, including diarrhoea and constipation
● Pinkish-red or bluish-red spots on the skin, which fade after about a week
● Skin rash or itching after bathing
● Dizziness
● Visual disturbances

If you experience what you believe are symptoms, do have your fluoride levels tested (see Resources Directory). Also reduce your intake of tea and soft drinks which are high in fluoride and drink herbal tea made with non-fluoridated water instead. Switch to non-fluoridated toothpaste and **never** let children use adult fluoride toothpaste. A poor diet only serves to increase your susceptibility to symptoms of fluoride poisoning. Adequate levels of magnesium, zinc and iron will help your body counter the affects of fluoride. Watch your consumption of prepared foods especially frozen vegetables which are high in fluoride. **Never use fluoridated water for baby formulae.**

• NUTRIENTS – THE WHOLE PICTURE •

Nutrients can best be described as the various properties contained in the food that we eat to nourish our bodies. Food contains vital elements, that do everything from building our bones, muscles and nerves to helping us create a new bloodstream every few months. These nutrients also play a fundamental role in the chemical and hormonal balance of our body and keep our entire metabolism regulated.

Most people in the West have minor deficiencies in many of these nutrients and have an overload of others such as fat and protein. A situation which is exclusive to our so called civilised cultures is that we experience illness due to the **lack** of certain nutrients and we can be malnourished even while we are overweight.

Medical science has been trying to understand nature since its conception but as far as nutrition is concerned its ignorance remains abysmal. Modern science continues to discover new nutrients and is constantly putting the pieces of the puzzle together, a puzzle we naturopaths feel should be left in a box. A classic example of this is vitamin C. A cure for scurvy, which is the final debilitating result of vitamin C deficiency and which manifests itself with bleeding gums, haemorrhages and extreme debility, was not properly understood by our ancestors. As early as 1602, John Manningham recorded a remedy which included scurvy grass and watercress, both high in vitamin C. Jacques Cartier visited Newfoundland for the second time in 1535 and landed with 100 out of his 103 crew prostrate with scurvy. A native among his men introduced him to a decoction of the leaves and bark of sassafras which restored all of his men to good health in only six days. By the eighteenth century it was finally understood that lemons and limes contain a substance we now call vitamin C which combats scurvy, hence the word 'limey' for British sailors who were given limes or lemons to eat on long voyages.

I remember when I first began to study nutrition many people just took vast amounts of vitamin C in its denatured isolated form, ascorbic acid. Medical nutritionists insisted this was the safe thing to do to make sure you were getting enough. Then it was discovered that vitamin C had a **complex**, rather like vitamin B. A complex is basically a vitamin or non-vitamin nutrient that is associated with one particular vitamin which must be present with it for complete assimilation and balance of nutrition. Some of the vitamin C complexes are rutin, hesperivin and bioflavonoids. When this was acknowledged, manufacturers started making vitamin C complex by adding these three nutrients. It was later discovered that the vitamin C complex was not used efficiently by our body unless calcium was present. So now the manufacturers added calcium to their synthetic cocktail. My point is this: the so-called nutrition experts now say this complex is complete, but they have been saying this all along. If, on the other hand, from the beginning, you ignored the scientific nutrition information and simply ate one orange every day, you would receive not only the RDA of vitamin C but also its complex components. Better still you would receive parts of the vitamin C complex that science hasn't discovered yet.

Another aspect of nutritional therapy that has been popular for very many years now is mega (meaning very large) doses of vitamins and minerals. This idea of 'if a little is good a lot must be better' is a dangerous one. Its proponents would go to extreme lengths with megadoses of nutrients most, I suspect, to avoid the horror of eating a Brussels sprout. Mega doses of **any** isolated nutrient outside and alienated from its natural wholefood environment can be dangerous. Certainly, anyone can see, smell and feel the difference if in your right hand you hold a fresh strawberry or orange and in your left you hold an ascorbic acid tablet. It doesn't take a genius to come to the conclusion that the fresh fruit has more vitality. Even if the ascorbic acid pill had ten times the vitamin C content, which one would your digestive system know how to work with?

THE REAL THING

It was Simeon Kirlian who discovered that all living things shine with a visible light that can be photographed. In other words there is a quantity of vital energy stored alongside the chemical structure of any living thing and as soon as food is cut, cooked or damaged in any way this vital energy begins to leak away from it. The vital energy contained in raw food grown in the best possible non chemicalised conditions is about as far away from synthetically manufactured vitamins as it is possible to be. So eating whole organic foods at the peak of their maturity will give you all the vitamins and minerals found in that food in their most vital forms and besides this they will also be in the right dose and proportion to one another. **There is no other place, besides foods, where these nutrients can be found in precisely this way**.

Whenever you find a vitamin or mineral in a natural food you will also find the other nutrient necessary to digest it in that same food. A true biochemical simply cannot exist by itself. It cannot be isolated and still be a natural substance.

The higher the dose of the substance the more that substance tends to take on the affects of a chemical drug. Ascorbic acid for example when taken in high doses can change the acidity of the body as a whole and so change the reactions of other biochemical processes which can be dangerous. In other words it forces your body to change chemically rather than letting it act as it would do naturally. It is wise to remember that as far as vitamins and minerals are concerned, as is the case with protein, *more is not better*. Excessive amounts of vitamins A, D, B_6 and iron can be toxic to both mother and baby.

MINERALS DEAD OR ALIVE

Another important consideration as far as nutrients are concerned is their source. It amazes me that millions of people dutifully swallow vitamins, minerals and other nutrient supplements every day and never stop to ask the question, 'What exactly are these substances made from?' People are very much mistaken if they assume they are manufactured from fruits, wholegrains and vegetables. The real source of these nutrients is appalling. Ninety-nine per cent of all vitamins sold are made from disgusting and toxic substances such as bacteria-laden oils collected from the liver of fish and petrochemicals. Most mineral supplements sold are hard-mined minerals.

They are basically rock. Just because we smash these rocks up into a fine powder does not mean we can even begin to digest them, and overdoses can be toxic, even fatal. A good example is iron. If you take too much iron in its raw form (such as iron supplements, tonics and pills) the side affects may begin with vomiting and abdominal cramping and quickly graduate to vomiting blood, hyperventilation, followed by coma and death in *less than two hours*. Many children have been poisoned by swallowing adult iron formulas. Have you ever heard of any children who died from eating too many beets? The point to understand here is that *raw* minerals from the earth are indigestible and about as helpful as swallowing an iron nail. Even if you grind it to iron filings, you still cannot digest it. So science alters the iron to make it digestible and by fooling nature, creates a potentially very dangerous product.

Some of the vitamin B complexes come from even stranger sources. The respected Merck's manual lists B_{12} as being cultivated on human faecal matter or from ground-up cows' livers already overloaded with steroids, antibiotics and insecticides. I kid you not! In natural healing we not only object to ingesting substances like this but we know we cannot eat rocks, so we let plant life do this job for us. We let plants dig their roots deep down into the soil, they ingest these crude minerals, assimilate them with the power of their green blood (chlorophyll) and sunlight. They then transmute these minerals into their own cell structures. By eating the plants we can now easily digest these plant minerals without any fear of side affects and toxic overdose. These minerals are now being presented to us by courtesy of the earth through nature's mediators – plants.

VITAMIN B_{12}

Lets scotch the B_{12} scare as far as vegans are concerned once and for all. As a vegan myself I am tired of this battered and inaccurate myth being thrown at me. This vitamin is necessary for normal blood-cell growth and nerve function. It is needed only in tiny amounts, an average of three millionths of a gram every day is sufficient for all adults, whether pregnant or not, and proportionately less for children. The liver is able to store a *three to five year supply* of vitamin B_{12}, and this acts as a great B_{12} buffer for the body. Consequently there is absolutely no need to ingest the vitamin daily. Consuming vitamin B_{12} in its active form (cyanocobalamin) every few days or even once a week is more than enough.

No animal makes B_{12}. It is made by bacteria that grow in the soil and in fermented food. B_{12} is only found in cow's liver and other flesh foods because that cow has eaten plants that have B_{12} bearing soil particles clinging to them, as well as having consumed water containing the bacterially made vitamins. The vitamin B_{12} the cow eats is stored in the cow's liver and muscles. It is true that to obtain B_{12} one can kill a cow and eat the liver and muscles. However there are gentler less expensive sources for humans to obtain this nutrient.

Practising vegans who do not believe in vitamin supplements, like myself, seldom become deficient in B_{12} because they obtain it from subtle but important sources:

1. There are bacteria within the human body that make vitamin B_{12} in the mouth, saliva, in the liver's bile, and within the intestinal contents. Some vegans may absorb the products of these natural vitamin generators that live within their own digestive system. So these people may internally meet their own B_{12} requirements and have absolutely no need of deriving it from any type of diet.
2. The diet of today's vegans usually includes food that has been fortified with B_{12} such as enriched cereals, soya milks, soya-based meat analogues

and nutritional yeast. The pregnant woman that is utilising these four to five products regularly should feel more than confident that she is satisfying her need for that vitamin.

3. B_{12} is present in virtually all sprouted seeds, particularly alfalfa. It is also very high in many herbs including comfrey, garlic, parsley and some superfoods such as spirulina and chlorella. If we maintain optimum intestinal health, particularly as far as producing the benign intestinal flora is concerned, our small intestines are capable of manufacturing their own B_{12}. Fermented food such as tempeh, miso and shoyu are also generally rich in B_{12}.

If you have any worries about this at all a simple blood test can determine whether your B_{12} level is adequate (hypersegmented white blood cells, or a vitamin B_{12} level below 150 picogrammes/ml are medical indications for B_{12} supplementation).

BIOCHEMICAL INDIVIDUALITY

Having said all this our own biochemical uniqueness has to be taken into account. Every human being differs in their ability to digest, assimilate and to metabolise foods. We differ in the chemical structure of our enzymes and we differ in the efficiency of our enzyme systems. We also differ in our nutritional requirements. Dr Roger Williams, who has done an enormous amount of work on biochemical individuality, discovered that in animals the requirements of a specific essential nutrient substance can vary by as much as ten times. While one animal might thrive on 1 mg of vitamin C daily another of the same species might need 16 mg in order to thrive. Recent studies in the requirement of essential fatty acids for males have suggested that they need three times more than females do. But I suspect further studies will show that the range of optimum amounts of essential fatty acids will show a similar spread to that already shown by other essential nutrients, perhaps tenfold or more. Conditions of stress, illness, factors in the diet such as sugar and saturated fatty acids may also increase the amount of essential nutrients needed. This may explain in part why so many experts have come up with widely diverging daily requirements for various nutrients. The Government's RDA is, in my opinion, ridiculously low. There has been a recent scare about synthetic vitamin A. And again this brings me back to my point. If nutrients are taken as nature intended in their natural balance in food it is impossible to hurt yourself with them. In addition to which you are ingesting hidden micro-nutrients that science has yet to discover and which are essential for our continuing good health.

CRAVINGS

It may well be that nutritional deficiencies lead to cravings or repulsions for certain foods. But each individual woman will be different. My feeling is that a healthy woman will allow nature to dictate her needs during pregnancy as far as food is concerned. If she starts to eat very peculiar things like coal, which I have known some pregnant women to do, this is because she is extremely mineral deficient. So such odd cravings need to be investigated. Most pregnant women I know start to go on benders on oatmeal porridge or kippers or fresh fruit, none of which if taken in excess will do you terrible amounts of harm. I presume they do this simply because the body has need of nutrients of this particular food.

VITAMIN B COMPLEX

So far scientists have discovered eleven components that go to make up the vitamin B complex but I can guarantee that many more besides this will be discovered in time. The B vitamins have many functions during pregnancy including a responsibility for foetal growth and cell division, your own digestion of protein and carbohydrate and the prevention of anaemia and possibly pre-eclampsia. In general terms the B vitamin complex helped to prevent nervousness, skin problems and lack of energy. Women who rely on processed and enriched breads, flours and rice for their B vitamins should remember that only thirteen of the eleven so far discovered are put back in after the milling process.

FOLIC ACID

Since 1991 women planning to become pregnant have been advised by the government to take supplements of folic acid but it is richly present in dark green leafy vegetables, organic nutritional yeast and dates. Ample helpings of broccoli and dark green leafy vegetables like spinach as well as one or two dried dates every few days will ensure the recommended 1 mg daily intake through pregnancy.

VITAMIN B$_6$

Excessive Vitamin B$_6$ can be toxic to mother and foetus so a total of 50 mg of B$_6$ per day should not be exceeded unless under the guidance of an orthomolecular therapist. B$_6$ in its natural form is present in green vegetables, grains, pulses and organic nutritional yeast. It is essential for vital energy producing reactions as well as healthy nerves and mucus membranes.

VITAMIN C

Vitamin C helps to produce flexible bloodcell walls (one of its components, the bioflavonoids, are particularly responsible for this), strong teeth and bones, a healthy immune system and a durable placenta during pregnancy. If you bruise easily or have bleeding gums you should take more vitamin C in your diet during your pregnancy. Smoking, stress and illness all increase the need for vitamin C because it is water soluble and therefore cannot be stored in the tissues.

Very importantly, vitamin C markedly increases the absorption of iron from the food into the body. For example 60 mg of vitamin C increases the absorption of iron in corn by five times, so vitamin C-containing foods like the tops of turnips, broccoli, Brussels sprouts, potatoes and sweet potatoes, peppers, tomatoes and cabbage are particularly effective combined with iron rich foods. Of course citrus fruits contain large amounts of vitamin C and vitamin C is also present in melons, strawberries, cauliflower, parsley, rosehips, kiwi and other exotic fruits. It is destroyed by contact with heat and air and therefore if not eating these foods raw, steam them and keep the container covered during cooking or bake them.

VITAMIN D

Vitamin D is not really a true vitamin. It is a hormone made within our own bodies. It is composed when sunlight touches our skin and activates a fatty substance called ergosterol. The ergosterol is transformed into active vitamin D and as it flows into the bloodstream through the walls of the small intestine, it enables us to absorb calcium from our food into our bloodstream. So vitamin D is closely connected with a calcium balance throughout the body, in the blood, in the bones and in the muscles.

Sunlight is so effective in creating vitamin D that fifteen minutes of walking outside simply exposing the face and arms is all that is required to meet our daily needs. Vitamin D is stored in the liver so a summer of gentle sunshine and moderate exposure to it should create all the body's vitamin D supplies and certainly enough to carry it throughout the winter. If brief daily sun exposure is possible there is no need even to ingest vitamin D in our food.

I will admit that for a pregnant woman living in a very cold climate, adequate sunlight exposure in winter can be a real problem. In this instance try to walk outside each day or if this is impossible at least sit near an open window. 400 IUs of vitamin D daily is more than adequate for a pregnant woman. Excessive **synthetic** vitamin D can be toxic to the mother and the developing foetus. Vitamin D-enriched soya milks are available and can be included in the diet as a dairy substitute but it is also possible, if you are still drinking milk, to find milk with added vitamin D.

VITAMIN E

If a woman is unable to get pregnant or is constantly having miscarriages I will often suspect a vitamin E deficiency among other things. Statistically 75 per cent of all pregnancies are aborted within the first thirty days and this is because if a woman is deficient in vitamin E the egg can be fertilised but the uterus cannot support the right environment for the pregnancy to continue onwards. Vegetables that are rich in vitamin E include watercress, spinach, lettuce, molasses, pulses, linseed, celery, parsley and turnip leaves. The highest source of all is wheatgerm oil but all oils can quickly go rancid and you can detect this by smelling an earthy odour. So wheatgerm oil should be stored in a dark container in the refrigerator. You can assimilate your food more thoroughly and efficiently if you include vitamin E in your meals and this in turn helps your baby get better use of the food you eat too. It is necessary for the proper development and function of the nervous system and helps the thyroid to work properly as well as the circulatory system.

• IMPORTANT MINERALS •

IRON

The need for iron during pregnancy escalates greatly simply because the mother and baby are busy creating large quantities of new blood. Whereas a non-pregnant woman requires 18 mg per day, a pregnant woman's need can go as high as 42 mg per day. There are also huge differences among women in the efficiency with which they absorb iron from the intestine into the bloodstream. That is some women absorb into their bloodstream a large fraction of the iron made in food and some much smaller amounts. On average most women absorb 10 per cent of the iron they consume. Remember that dairy produce actually inhibits the absorption of iron. The use of dairy products also crowds out greens and other iron-rich plant foods. Women who are good absorbers of iron should get sufficient supplies from green leafy vegetables, raisins, wholegrains and foods made from wholegrains, nuts, seeds, pulses, molasses and dried fruits. Please note vitamin C hugely increases the absorption of iron from the food into the body so green leafy vegetables (which are abundant in both iron and vitamin C) are especially valuable foods during pregnancy. Sixty mg of vitamin C increases the absorption of iron in corn by five times. So vitamin C-containing foods such as broccoli, Brussels sprouts, potatoes, sweet potatoes, peppers, tomatoes and cabbage are especially good to combine with iron-rich foods.

So the prevention, detection and treatment of anaemia differs for each woman depending on her efficiency of absorption of iron. It is difficult and unwise to try and adhere to an iron-clad rule about supplements for every woman. Excessive iron taken in its *synthetic* form can cause stomach irritation and actually be toxic to both the mother and baby.

1. Eat plenty of the iron and vitamin C foods listed above.
2. Make sure you go to your pre-natal check-ups and foster good communication and co-operation with your health-care practitioner.
3. I always determine, if possible, my pregnant client's haemoglobin levels at the beginning of their pregnancy, and check the levels every four to eight weeks or more frequently if necessary as the pregnancy progresses. If the haemoglobin value stays above 14 gms/dl, and the pregnant client is staying in positive iron balance on her dietary intake alone, I will not recommend any additional supplementation. A fall of the haemoglobin towards 12 dl concerns me and I will begin by suggesting a delicious juice made of two thirds carrot juice with one third beetroot juice and a half inch piece of fresh ginger root to add a sparkle to the taste and facilitate digestion. Only if this proves inadequate will I then go on to suggest superfoods such as Spirulina and Chlorella.

THE CALCIUM MYTH

Many people drink milk believing it to be high in calcium but most milk is pasteurised, homogenised, or processed and denatured in some way which degrades the calcium in it. This makes the calcium content almost impossible to utilise.

A pregnant woman has a particularly high need of calcium but what most people don't understand is calcium's role in the body. It is needed for the healthy function of muscle, blood and bone in both the mother and foetus, but one of its most vital functions is to neutralise acid in the system. All dairy products except butter are extremely acid forming. So you're trapped in a vicious circle here. People eating dairy products for calcium are utilising the existing calcium in their systems to neutralise the affects of the dairy products they are eating!

The good news is that calcium is found in all foods that grow in the ground especially green leafy vegetables, tofu from soya beans, all legumes (beans, peas, lentils, chick peas, etc.), carrots, sesame seeds and its butter, sunflower seeds, and all nuts, nut milks and nut butters are super abundant in calcium. All these sources are easily digested because they have an excellently balanced calcium/phosphorus ratio, that is their phosphorus content is much higher than their calcium content.

THE SYNERGY OF CALCIUM

The body's ability to absorb calcium is directly dependent on the amount of phosphorus in the diet. It seems the lower the ratio of phosphorus the greater the loss of bone density. The higher the calcium/phosphorus ratio the less the bone loss and the stronger the skeletal structure, always assuming the amount of protein in the diet is not excessive. Foods where the phosphorus ratio is low and therefore calcium is least available are – you've guessed it – meat and fish. Magnesium is also essential for the proper assimilation of calcium in the ratio of five for calcium to three of magnesium and yes! I can see you are getting ahead of me here, all the plant foods previously mentioned have this in perfect ratio.

Pregnant women need 1,000 mg of calcium daily. To give you a graphic idea of how much easier it is to assimilate this from plant sources, if you were to draw the calcium/phosphorous ratio in cabbage it would represent the World Trade Centre compared to the equivalent in chicken livers which would represent just a small four-drawer chest.

HOW TO GET OPTIMAL CALCIUM IN PREGNANCY

1. Cut down on flesh foods, fish and dairy products.
2. Ensure three servings of plant-based sources daily, for example: 8 fl oz (225 ml) carrot juice, a cup of broccoli and 2 level tablespoons of tahini. This will ensure you have the requisite 1000 mg of calcium daily needed in pregnancy.

3. Save the water in which you cook or steam your vegetables and add it to soups, sauces and salad dressings because some calcium may be leached into the water.
4. Keep your protein intake low (see page 27).
5. Some nutritionists are concerned that all the calcium that is eaten may not be absorbed from the intestine into the bloodstream as it can be bound to other substances in plant material such as oxalic or phytic acid. They worry that the amount of usable calcium might be less than the amounts listed in nutritional tables for vegetables high in oxalic acid including spinach, cashews and almonds. Fortunately this calcium-inhibiting effect is theoretical rather than real as calcium deficiency from inadequate dietary intake is actually quite rare under these circumstances. Apparently, on a vegan diet based on whole plant foods containing only moderate protein and calcium, the human intestine actually becomes more efficient at absorbing calcium, but just to be absolutely certain use the greens that are rich in calcium and relatively free of oxilic or phytic acid and root vegetables. The best usable calcium providers are broccoli, mustard and cress, turnips, celery, lettuce and all root vegetables.

Calcium rich herbal tea

2 parts oat straw
1 part alfalfa
1 part nettles

1 part peppermint
1 part horse tail
4 parts raspberry leaf

Place 1 oz (30 g) of herbs in cold water and bring to a simmer over a low heat. Remove from the heat source immediately and keep the pot covered for 20 minutes or longer before straining and drinking. Aim to drink three large breakfast cups a day, sweeten if desired.

MAGNESIUM

Magnesium deficiencies can easily be confused with calcium ones because they have similar symptom patterns. One way to tell the difference between the two is that a magnesium deficiency usually manifests itself more acutely. Magnesium gives bones and teeth their strength while calcium provides the structure. Without magnesium bones would not support the skeletal frame and the teeth would become brittle. Magnesium causes the stomach's secretion of hydrochloric acid to diminish so it can inhibit calcium absorption because calcium requires an acidic medium for proper assimilation. The general rule for magnesium is to get twice as much calcium as magnesium but not to go over 400 mg of magnesium in any one day. An excess of magnesium can cause diarrhoea.

Good dietary sources of magnesium include nuts, soya beans, all leafy green vegetables and sprouted seeds, chicory, beet tops, figs, apples, lemons and peaches. Whole grains, particularly brown rice and all the seeds are also rich in magnesium.

ZINC

Zinc is certainly essential for the foetus as it is responsible for the formulation of RNA and DNA as well as the health of the pregnant mother. Fortunately it is found in wholegrains, green leafy vegetables, mushrooms, nuts, seeds (especially sesame/tahini and sprouted seeds), pulses, tofu, miso, wheatgerm and organic nutritional yeast. These foods should more than adequately meet all your body's needs for zinc. A deficiency in zinc can easily be detected by white spots appearing on the nails.

If all this talk of vitamins and minerals is throwing you into a blind panic please remember that women have been giving birth and raising happy healthy babies long before vitamin and mineral supplements were ever invented. Ideally, fresh locally grown organic produce cultivated in healthy fertile soil is the best way of ensuring a natural balance of nutrients in the diet. If you eat steamed green and yellow vegetables on a daily basis as well as a nice large green salad that includes fresh dark leaves, a few carrots and a strip of dulse (or other sea vegetable for trace minerals), all your vitamin and mineral needs should be met adequately and deliciously.

VITAMINS

Water Soluble (not stored, needed daily)	Fat Soluble (stored in your liver, needed three to five times per week)
B complex including B_1, B_2, B_6, choline, biotin, folic acid, the rest of the B complex and vitamin C	Vitamin A, vitamin E, essential fatty acids
Found in:	Found in:
Green vegetables including alfalfa, sprouts, avocados, green beans, broccoli, Brussels sprouts, cabbage, cucumber, chicory, leeks, mustard greens, peppers, lettuce, spinach and the dark green leafy tops of any root vegetables. Organic nutritional yeast. Fruits including melons of all sorts and citrus fruits. Wholegrains.	Yellow vegetables and oil-rich foods including carrots, corn, pumpkin, all the squashes, sweet potatoes, corn oil, linseed, sunflower and seeds. Wholegrains.

The average non-pregnant woman requires 44 g of protein a day, 800 mg of calcium and 18 mg of iron. The average pregnant woman requires an additional 30 g of protein, 400 mg of calcium and a total of 60 mg of iron.

• SUPERFOODS •

PHYTOCHEMICALS

These are the biologically active chemicals found in all natural foods. Scientists are only just beginning to wake up to their importance. They contribute to the biochemistry of the body with as much weight as vitamins and minerals do. So far fifteen phytochemicals have been identified but as with all pioneering scientific research you can be assured many more will be uncovered in future years. They include chlorophyll, coumarins, enzymes, flavenoids, indoles, lignans, phenols, phytoestrogens, allium compounds, plant sterols, inhibitors of protease and saponins. All of these phytochemicals are richly present in herbs.

CHLOROPHYLL

Green foods are rich in phytochemicals. All plant life depends upon the sun. We depend upon those plants. Sunlight activates the green chlorophyll in plants to generate energy for the plants. Molecules of chlorophyll are constructed around magnesium and carry oxygen around the inside of plant cells which in turn creates energy for the plant. It is this stored energy in plants which we eat and absorb to sustain us. Plant energy is the primary energy of life because even carnivores eat animals which eat plants.

Our vitality depends upon a good supply of oxygen and germs will gravitate towards tissue which is oxygen deficient.

The advantages of taking chlorophyll

All grasses contain fresh chlorophyll as do phyto-planktons such as chlorella and spirulina. There was a village in Austria during the Second World War which had all its food supplies commandeered by invading troops. The population was consequently forced to live off grass. Not only did the villagers thrive but many of their degenerative diseases began to heal completely. While you might blanch at the thought of eating grass, the good news is that other dark green vegetables such as spinach, cabbage and nettles also contain large amounts of chlorophyll as, of course, does chlorella.

The CGF factor noted in chlorella is also present in wheat and barley grass. To obtain all its benefits it must be administered orally or as a rectal injection and must be freshly made. Synthetic chlorophyll won't do and can be poisonous.

BARLEY AND WHEAT GRASSES

Barley and wheat grasses can be sprouted and the sprouts are more potent nutritionally than the grains themselves, being richly abundant with vitamins minerals and chlorophyll. Barley is twice as rich in protein as wheat. Both grasses can be juiced and the juice is extremely beneficial. Pregnant women may find wheat and barley grass in their juiced form makes them feel nauseous. Try it, but if you find it too difficult to get down leave it. You could try it instead in its dried, superfood form.

Wheat grass juice.

The simplest and most natural way to obtain wheat grass juice is to chew small amounts of grass, then swallow only the juice. It is best to use a manual juicer designed especially for grass because its slow rotation prevents oxidation of the juice. These are available from the Holistic Research Company (see Resources Directory). (The use of a blender or centrifugal juice extractor oxidises the juice which greatly reduces its nutritional value.)

Simply feed the grass into the receptable and the juice will flow out of the spout. The machine ejects the dry pulp and it need only be cleaned once per day.

Let the juice sit for a few minutes after juicing so that the sediment settles in the bottom of the glass. Do not drink the sediment.

Mixing sprouted seeds, celery, parsley or spinach with wheat grass makes the juice more palatable but use small quantities of the grass during each feeding of the machine. One box of wheat grass, which is properly planted and cared for, can produce up to 2½ lbs (1.1 kg) of grass, and 1 lb (454 g) of seeds will produce about 4 lb (1.8 kg) of grass. With the correct grass juicer it is possible to extract at least 8 fl oz (2 z 5 ml) of juice from 1 lb (454 g) of grass. Harvesting should begin between the seventh and fourteenth day of planting.

Growing your own wheat grass

Obtain two large, heavy-duty plastic bin bags and fill one with the best available compost. Add more compost to a plastic tray 9 × 5 × 2 ins (30 × 13 × 50 cm) or thereabouts and then sprinkle some crushed kelp with your fingertips on to the soil and mix it in well. Plant the wheat seed shallowly, lightly covering it with soil and put the tray into the bin bag which will create a greenhouse effect. Keep the tray in a window and after three days remove the covering.

Somewhere between the seventh and fourteenth day the grass will be at least 7 inches (18 cm) high and ready to harvest. After the first harvest the second growth of wheat grass is still worthwhile, but the third growth is of little value.

After harvesting the grass, store the sod in the second plastic bin bag by placing the first mat root downwards and all the other roots upwards. Then drop a few earth worms into this, closing the bag very loosely so that the worms are able to breathe. In three to six weeks the sod will break down into soil which can again be used for planting.

When using wheat or barley grass juice for the first time it is a good idea to take it in very small quantities, perhaps only a tablespoon. Take enough to make you feel uncomfortable but not so much that you feel like vomiting it up again. Both are powerful cleansers because of their high enzyme content, so they will start immediate reactions with toxins and mucus in the stomach, often causing nausea. This feeling of nausea merely proves that they are needed and should be taken regularly. Thirty minutes before drinking any of the juice, drink a quarter of a lemon squeezed into a glass of water or, if you have an acid stomach, a glass of mint tea. Both methods will clean out mucus from the stomach and minimise discomfort.

Grass juices in 1 or 2 fl oz (30 or 60 ml) doses can be taken immediately before sprouted seeds. Try to take any grass juice on an empty or nearly empty stomach. That way it is immediately absorbed. Diluted or undiluted rectal implants of wheat grass juice can be used and are often much easier to absorb than taking it orally. The correct amount for a rectal implant is 4 fl oz (120 ml). Use 1 or 2 fl oz (30 or 60 ml) of pure wheat grass juice diluted with 2 fl oz (60 ml) of purified water. Raw grass juices can be used as a mouthwash. Remember chlorophyll will bring oxygen to the mouth and this is particularly helpful for anyone who has thrush or candida in their mouth or throat.

The easiest way to ensure you have plenty of chlorophyll in your diet is to eat a regular helping every day of phytoplantons or sprouted seeds which have green leaves attached to them.

ENZYMES

Some of the phytochemicals in foods are more potent if eaten raw. Dr Max Bircher-Benner, a Swiss nutritionist and a visionary before his time, understood this long before science had proved it. 'Mangez-vivant!' he would say to his patients, meaning, 'Eat living food.' He had no objections to eating meat as long as it was uncooked and in its entirety of blood, fat, bones, entrails, skin and flesh. In other words, exactly the way a lion eats prey in the wilderness. And how many of us will be willing to do that? He understood that as soon as any food was processed in some way it altered the state of the whole food energy and produced ill health. A more acceptable and appetising way to enjoy raw foods is to eat plants. We have the ability to protect the delicate enzymes in such food as it passes through our digestive tracts so that about 70 per cent reaches the colon intact. By binding with oxygen enzymes enhance the activity of our intestinal flora. Too much oxygen in the digestive tract encourages putrefaction and intestinal toxemia and such fermentation has long been linked with all sorts of degenerative diseases including digestive cancers. Foods which are massively rich in enzymes include freshly sprouted seeds, grains and pulses, papaya, pineapples, and fermented foods such as sauerkraut and rejuvelac, the water collected off soaked wheat before it is sprouted.

ALLIUM COMPOUNDS

The most famous member of the Allium family is undoubtedly garlic, but it also embraces leeks, chives, spring onions, shallots and onions. Their main active ingredients are sulphur compounds including allixin, allicin, diallyl trisulphid and diallyl disulphid.

GARLIC

The ancient Egyptians, Greeks and Romans all used garlic copiously to increase strength and fight disease and illness. Hippocrates used garlic specifically to treat cancer. In the First World War the British government used garlic in the battlefield hospitals. It saved thousands of lives. It was used in numerous preparations to disinfect and heal battle wounds internally. Garlic was also administered to treat typhoid fever and dysentery.

Today garlic is the leading over-the-counter drug in numerous European and Asian countries. It is an official drug in many countries and prescribed by medical doctors outside the US for hypertension (high blood pressure), high cholesterol, cancer, and as a broad spectrum antibiotic, antiviral agent and fungicide.

Garlic is famous for its healing power with heart disease. Countries where garlic consumption is high have a lower incidence of heart disease than average. Garlic lowers serum cholesterol and triglyceride levels and reduces the build up of atherosclerotic plaque in our arteries. It does this partly by increasing the blood levels of high density lipo-proteins (HDLs). These lipoproteins clear the blood of excess cholesterol and fat. Garlic also lowers low density lipoproteins (LDLs) which can attribute to arterial plaque. Medical researchers have also found substances in garlic that inhibit blood platelet aggregation (the sticking together of blood cells). Because of its powerful effect on blood pressure, the Japanese Food and Drug Administration has approved garlic and it is now an official drug listed in the Japanese Pharmacopoeia.

Garlic is an effective cancer therapy. One third of all the medical research into garlic is cancer related. The National Cancer Institute has found that cancer incidence worldwide is lowest in the countries where garlic consumption is reported to be the highest. Garlic has been shown to help white blood cells combat cancer and increase the ability to destroy tumours. When the properties of garlic are present in the bloodstream, many aspects of our immunity system are enhanced. Garlic helps to stimulate interferon production, enhance natural killer cells, stop tumour growth, and even reduce the associated pain of cancer. Garlic has been found in double blind studies to reduce the incidence of colon-rectal cancer and stomach cancer. In one medical university study garlic reduced stomach cancer ten times more effectively than in those who did not eat garlic. With over eighty different sulphur compounds, it is a free radical scavenger. This is just another way that garlic protects from cancer, even those that are chemically induced.

Garlic juice diluted one part in 125,000 has been found to inhibit the growth of bacteria and destroys both gram positive and gram negative bacteria making it a broad spectrum antibiotic. Garlic used as an antibacterial agent in Russia is so revered it has been christened Russian penicillin. Unlike antibiotics garlic is totally selective in its bacteria destruction, only killing bacteria that's harmful to our body. What is thrilling is that at the same time garlic actually enhances our friendly bacteria and improves our intestinal flora and digestion.

Some say that the reason you don't catch colds when you eat garlic is because no one will come near you! Garlic is certainly a powerful antiviral agent. Many feel it's the cure for the common cold. It will destroy the different viruses that cause upper respiratory infections and influenza. Garlic has been shown to destroy on contact the viral infections of measles, mumps, mononucleosis, chicken pox, herpes simplex 1 and 2, herpes zoster, viral hepatitis, scarlet fever, rabies and others.

Garlic's antifungal ability is second to none. Laboratory tests have proved to be more potent than any known antifungal agent including Nystatin. Garlic will regulate the overgrowth of Candida albicans, and indeed it goes far further than this because it actively encourages the growth of benign intestinal flora in the colon.

FURTHER HIDDEN GOODNESS

The indoles and isothyocyanats (ITCs) are richly present in broccoli, Brussels sprouts, cabbage, cauliflower, cress, kale, horseradish, kohlrabi, mustard, radish and turnip. ITCs are now known to prevent colon cancer and if you eat at least a serving of cabbage a week you have 66 per cent more of a chance of avoiding cancer than people who never eat cabbage. Indoles actually activate the detoxification processes of the body. Indeed they go further and accelerate the body's ability to deactivate the particular oestrogen that can promote breast cancer. The optimal dose is 10 oz (280 g) of these vegetables every week steamed or raw. So everything your mum told you about eating up your greens now turns out to be true! The organic oxilic acid found in raw green leafy vegetables is excellent for treating constipation, but once cooked, the oxilic acid can settle in the joints, so if you are prone to gout or rheumatism don't eat your greens cooked. As long ago as the 1950s the British Ministry of Health and Public Service Laboratory accepted that spinach juice, cabbage juice, kale and parsley juices were far superior to milk for relieving excess production of hydrochloric acid in the stomach and as this can be a problem in the last trimester of pregnancy do mix a little green juice with your other vegetable juices.

ROSEHIPS, ORANGE AND LEMON PEELS

These are some of the best sources of vitamin C and contain the whole vitamin C complex including bioflavonoids, rutin, hesperidin, calcium and all the trace elements that are now known to be necessary to assimilate vitamin C. All citrus peels contain pectin which are known to remove heavy metals such as mercury and lead from the body and even radioactive contamination like Strontium 90. So when you eat citrus fruit always eat some of the white pith with them.

BIOFLAVONOIDS

However the bioflavonoids in the pith of all citrus fruit is highly active and unstable and easily destroyed by heat and exposure to the air.

It has been appreciated for some years now that some of the bioflavonoids and particularly Quercitin are extremely active against viruses particularly herpes. Nobiletin is powerfully anti-inflammatory and the rutin richly present in the buckwheat lifts depression as well as acting as a preventative against bruising.

Certain bioflavonoids are believed to be anti-carcinogenic and the methoxylated bioflavonoid stops red blood cells clumping together decreasing blood viscosity by as much as 6 per cent.

All bioflavonoids are at their most powerful and active when the body is under stress and considering that many of them are useful for combating fungi, viruses and bacteria this is a particularly desirable asset.

NON-ACTIVE SACCHAROMYCES CEREVASIAE NUTRITIONAL YEAST

There are literally hundreds of different types of yeast that have various qualities. Saccharomyces cerevasiae is one of them, but many of the yeasts on the market today are the by-products of manufacturing processes in the brewing industry (hence the name brewers yeast) or designed for the baking industry. In the past some of these yeasts have been grown on rags and old newspapers. These yeasts are often used as food supplements. My feeling is that not only is their nutritional value suspect, their quality is very poor and some are even toxic. In this instance nature gives you a clue simply because they often taste and smell somewhat unpleasant and bitter. More importantly they are still active, meaning they are alive, and can be damaging to those people who have yeast infections and/or overgrowth problems with candida albicans.

Saccharomyces cerevasiae nutritional yeast is grown solely for human consumption as a nutritional food supplement. It is cultivated on a base of pure beet and cane molasses and it absorbs this base in the same way as plants utilise minerals in the soil. Molasses is used because it provides the yeast with an abundant organic source of B vitamins and minerals. Once the yeast is harvested it is thoroughly washed and dried. During the drying process it is heated just enough to stabilise, so making it completely non fermentable. This process not only makes the yeast incapable of any further fermentation in the digestive tract but helps it to be easily digested and assimilated. It is therefore particularly recommended for those with internal bacterial or fungal infections including candida albicans.

SPIRULINA

Spirulina has the highest protein content of any natural food (65 per cent or more) far more than animal and fish flesh (15–25 per cent), soyabeans (35 per cent), eggs (12 per cent), or whole milk (3 per cent). And 95 per cent of this protein is digestible. This is particularly important for those suffering from intestinal malabsorption (caeliacs, those affected by candida, Crohn's disease, mucous colitis and many people over forty who have dwindling supplies of hydrochloric acid in their stomachs or pregnant women in their last trimester who are finding it difficult to eat anything).

LIFE IN THE FAT LANE

Spirulina's fat content is only 5 per cent, far lower than almost any other protein source. Ten grammes (one tablespoon) has only 36 calories and virtually no cholesterol. So spirulina is a low-fat, low-calorie cholesterol-free source of protein. In contrast a large egg yields 300 mg (less than ¼ of an ounce) of cholesterol and eighty calories but only has as much protein as one tablespoon of spirulina.

COLON CLEANSING

Engevita nutritional yeast, chlorella and spirulina are the only forms of protein that are not mucoid forming in the intestines. Spirulina acts as a metabolic activator directly on the body's tissues at a cellular level promoting increased activity to burn up mucus-forming substances (such as the wastes from meat, eggs and dairy products). Spirulina acts as an aggressive cleansing herb that empties toxins out of the body tissues into the lymph and is a superb addition in both fasting and colon-cleansing programmes.

SPIRULINA AND HYPOGLYCAEMIA

The minimal amount of carbohydrate in spirulina, 15–25 per cent, consists of two polysaccharides which are easily absorbed by the body with minimum insulin intervention. Spirulina supplies rapid energy without taxing the pancreas so it will not precipitate hypoglycaemia. Indeed it is actively helpful for controlling the sweeping blood-sugar curves which so debilitate hypoglycaemics or women who become hypoglycaemic in pregnancy which is not uncommon. It is also the richest source of B_{12} in food. Higher than beef, liver, chlorella, or sea vegetables, so it is highly recommended in a vegan diet. It actually reduces cholesterol, triglyceride and LDL levels. This may be partially due to its unusual and very high gamma linoleic acid (GLA) content. One tablespoon of spirulina provides 100 mg of GLA and dietary GLA helps heart conditions, PMT, obesity and arthritis.

SPIRULINA AND DIGESTION

Spirulina actually encourages healthy lactobacillus by 327 per cent over a hundred days and increases the efficient absorption of Vitamin B_1 inside the caecum, the murkiest part of the colon most prone to encourage the breeding of parasites by 43 per cent. Healthy lactobacillus means that better digestion and absorption protects from infection and stimulates the immune system.

SPIRULINA AND ANAEMIA

The iron in spirulina is twice as absorbable as the iron found in vegetables and meat and it is therefore highly recommended for people prone to anaemia and for women in pregnancy. Spirulina was used to treat the one hundred and sixty thousand children suffering from radiation poisoning at Chernobyl. Remember that in addition to the toxic waste produced by nuclear power plants we are all constantly exposed to radiation from the atmosphere, leaking microwave ovens, electrical power lines, X-ray machines, illuminated neon signs, clock faces, garage door openers and frequent flying. Spirulina also inhibits the growth of bacteria, yeast and fungi which is why it is so important as part of the candida controlling programme and to heal internal bacterial infections. A diet of 30 per cent of spirulina has been shown to radically decrease the toxicity of inorganic mercury and chemical anodynes, antibiotics and anti-cancer drugs which can cause acute nephrotoxicity, that is poisons in the kidneys.

CHLORELLA

This is second only to spirulina in its nutritional content. Another of the blue/green algaes, the cell wall has to be artificially cracked to make the nutrients more available and increase its digestibility. So my first preference would always be for spirulina over chlorella simply because any substance which has had to be artificially messed about with takes it one step further away from nature. Having said this chlorella has some unique properties of its own. Whereas spirulina is a multi-cell, spiral-shaped plant which grows on salty or brackish water, chlorella is a round, single-cell algae which grows on fresh water. This means it contains five times as much chlorophyll as spirulina. It is also different from spirulina as it contains Chlorella Growth Factor (CGF). In a study conducted by Doctor Yoshio Yamagishi published in 1961 fifty ten-year-old students given 2 g of chlorella daily for 112 days outstripped their control group in height and weight over this period of time. Chlorella's capacity to stimulate growth in the young is probably due to its nucleic acid content of RNA and DNA, which are important building blocks for life. RNA and DNA accelerate growth in the young and help repair damaged tissue in adults.

It has been suggested that the loss of energy and physical deterioration associated with ageing is due to the increasing breakdown of DNA and RNA which are needed to keep the cells healthy. As we age our natural production of RNA and DNA becomes sluggish; this commences at about the age of twenty. A diet rich in DNA and RNA foods produces more energy and a more youthful appearance, and alleviates long-standing problems such as arthritis, memory loss and depression.

Spirulina and chlorella are excellent additions to your diet while pregnant, particularly during the first trimester when you may be suffering from morning sickness and therefore having an inadequate intake of concentrated nutrients. The colour of both may be a bit off-putting but if you mix them into a fruit smoothy (see page 35) they are easily digestible and if you sip the fruit smoothy with your eyes closed, who's to know?

• SUGAR •

Most people eat 5 oz (150g) of sugar daily; that is a phenomenal 120 lbs 54.4 kg yearly. Our endocrine systems are only designed to deal with a relatively slow absorption glucose naturally diluted in fruits or vegetables. Refined sugar gives the body a sugar rush, going straight into the bloodstream and raising the blood sugar level very fast. The pancreas rebalances the blood by removing the sugar into storage above the liver in the form of glucose. A high level of sugar will result in a trigger-happy pancreas, which seeps insulin at the slightest provocation. The body feels sluggish and constantly in need of a boost so the hypoglycaemic reaches for yet more sugar and becomes trapped in a vicious cycle as the blood sugar level pitches wildly up and down while the beleaguered pancreatic cells puff away in an effort to keep pace.

Sugar in its refined state is empty calories. It is 99.96 per cent sucrose and totally devoid of vitamin, minerals and enzymes. Professor John Yudkin called it, 'Pure, white and deadly.' Vitamins, minerals and enzymes are essential for the digestion, assimilation and utilisation of sugar, but analysis of molasses (the byproduct of sugar refining) shows six B vitamins and eight minerals which have been detached from the sugar. And these are just a portion of the nutrients the human body must somehow provide in order to metabolise sugar. The missing elements much be stolen from real food in the diet, from nutrients in the blood that are intended for other functions and from the reserve stored in our bones. Only in this way can the simple carbohydrate sugar initiate complex ones and act like a real food.

In sharp contrast, a carbohydrate which is a real food has its sugars accompanied by fibre, vitamins, minerals, enzymes, protein and fat, that is everything necessary to complete the metabolic activities that will be fired by sugar. Complex carbohydrates supply the body with a slow, steady stream of blood sugar and none of the essential components are missing. This is natural sugar metabolism. This is why eating refined sugar causes the bloodstream to leap and plunge dramatically. Sugar inhibits the ability of our white blood cells to destroy bacteria. A couple of teaspoons of sugar can undermine the strength of white blood cells by 25 per cent, so reducing our resistance to everything ranging from colds to cancer. A glass of cola contains about thirty-two teaspoons of sugar!

If you eliminate sugar from your diet you stand a good chance of reducing dental decay, helping weight control, improving digestion, improving and correcting various blood abnormalities involving fats, uric acid, glucose, the stickiness of blood platelets and regulating the production of insulin and cortisol.

The problem is most of us have a natural craving for sweet things. Perhaps encouraged by the sweetness of breast milk or because natural vitamins and minerals taste sweet, in the form of fresh or dried fruits and young crisp vegetables.

A good alternative to sugar is date sugar. It is a solid wholefood made of dates that have been pitted, dried and ground. It is suitable for sprinkling on foods but does not mix well or dissolve easily, so it can be a problem if used for baking and cooking. In this instance thinned honey or maple syrup is a better idea.

ARTIFICIAL SWEETENERS

Artificial sweeteners, many of which it is now suggested might be carcinogenic, **are not** a good sugar substitute. A few years ago Aspartame (the generic name for the chemical used in NutraSweet) was the subject of investigation about its effect on blood pressure and behaviour. A study carried out in Leeds in England on 95 volunteers aged 18 to 22 showed that people actually felt hunger after eating foods sweetened with Aspartame. This effect is not very desirable considering most people are using artificial sweeteners to lose weight or to stabilise their weight. You would have thought we might have learned our lesson by now with saccharine, which is now known to cause bladder cancer in rats and is sold with a commensurate warning. So I would strongly recommend you avoid artificial sweeteners altogether during pregnancy in all forms, no matter what their source.

Aspartame and phenylalanine may alter brain growth in the foetus. Marketed under the brand name of NutraSweet, my advice is that pregnant women should avoid it until more extensive testing has been done on its effects. So far no adverse effects have been documented but concern has been raised about the effects on the foetus and on children. Again, read the labels.

• SALT •

If you took everything in a supermarket, ground it all together and analysed the resulting powder, you would find approximately a ratio of ten parts sodium to one part potassium. If you then went out to a stretch of field or forest and ground the contents together the result would be, in inverse ratio, ten parts potassium to one of sodium. Salt is ubiquitously present in all sorts of foods including things you wouldn't suspect like beer, baking soda, cereals, dried, evaporated or tinned milk, cheese and custard powder. If you eat a typical English breakfast of cornflakes, eggs and bacon, and marmite and salted butter on toast you will have already consumed 1.5 g of salt, nearly half your daily requirement. Salt also appears in many of the 400 and more additives in our food (in the form of monosodium glutamate, sodium bicarbonate, sodium nitrate, sodium benzoate, sodium proportionate and sodium citrate) so it is not hard to imagine how we can rapidly ingest 1 oz (30 g) of salt a day.

The problem with salt is that in excess it pulls extra water with it, which expands the volume of blood. This makes the pressure increase inside the circulation, rather as adding more water to a filled water balloon would do, exerting more pressure on the balloon's walls. Blood pressure which is elevated by extra salt and water is called volume hypertension. Women with this type of hypertension will lower their pressure by avoiding salt and increasing water excrescence. In the body there is a fine balance of sodium and potassium and these act together to maintain the osmotic pressure in a state of equilibrium inside and outside the cells. Chemical diuretics tend to leach potassium out of the system upsetting the body's natural potassium/sodium balance and often necessitating the addition of a potassium substitute, part of the crazy knock-on effects of chemical medicine. I have already mentioned the damage diuretics can do to the body (see Appendix I).

The good news is that salt, which is a combination of two minerals, sodium and chloride, is found in perfect ratio in nearly all vegetables, especially carrots, celery, beets and olives; and sea vegetables are a particularly good source of sodium chloride as the salt is accompanied by abundant trace minerals including iodine held in solution in sea water.

Because sodium chloride is so widely distributed among natural foods, it is *never* nutritionally necessary to add salt to food. Salt in its natural form in vegetables is important in a pregnant woman's diet since it contributes to retention of water in body tissues which in turn builds a reserve of fluid to help sustain the increases. Salt is an acquired not an inborn taste. Remember 90 per cent of the salt you eat is actually hidden in food. All salt whether it be rock, sea or plain table salt has virtually the same chemical composition and sodium content, so there is absolutely no point in just switching to another kind because it sounds healthier.

SALT SUBSTITUTES

Salt substitutes containing potassium can be a problem for women with kidney disease or diabetes, and all salt substitutes as far as I know contain potassium chloride. Besides which, potassium chloride tastes very bitter when cooked for some time, and manufacturers suggest that it needs to be added at the end of cooking to avoid this. Far better, I feel, to unlearn our taste for salt and to use herbs, spices and garlic as flavouring. A good salt substitute, which I particularly like, is two parts of kelp powder mixed with one part of parsley, one part of garlic powder, one part of cayenne pepper and one part of marjoram. The Japanese make up an unusual salt mixture of toasted sesame meal mixed with a small portion of salt and I have adapted this replacing the salt with equal parts of cayenne pepper and garlic powder. The proportions are nine parts of sesame seed meal to one part each of cayenne and garlic. The sesame meal needs to be roasted until it is golden brown in a frying pan over a strong heat but without any fat whatsoever.

Simply stir it around with a wooden spoon until it is the right colour. Let it cool, grind it in a liquidiser and then add the correct proportions of cayenne and garlic. This is a milder flavouring than the one first mentioned.

• ADDITIVES, PRESERVATIVES AND INSECTICIDES •

One thousand million gallons of pesticides are now being used every year on British farms. The London Food Commission's report 'Food Adulteration and How to Beat It' states that of the 426 principle chemicals legally used in over 3,000 brands of pesticides and fertilisers, 164 of these have been implicated in causing cancer, genetic mutations, irritant reactions and reproductive problems ranging from impotence to birth defects. According to Friends of the Earth the record number of times a single lettuce has been sprayed may be as much as forty-six. The organochlorines, including DDT, are classified as 'persistent' simply because they are not easily destroyed or degraded. They are attracted to fatty substances and so can be found in greater amounts than elsewhere in milk and other dairy products, meat and human breast milk. While DDT itself has long been banned in the UK and the USA, other organochlorines are still used, in spite of animal and bacterial studies which have consistently linked them to cancer, birth defects and genetic mutations. In 1975 the Council on Environment Quality unequivocally stated that meat and dairy products account for over 95 per cent of the populations intake of DDT. The same percentage is true for the other pesticides:

> Meat contains approximately fourteen times more pesticides than do plant foods; dairy products five and a half times more. Thus, by eating foods of animal origin, one ingests greatly concentrated amounts of hazardous chemicals. Analysis of various foods by the FDA show that meat, poultry, fish, cheese and other dairy products contain levels of these pesticides more often and in greater amounts than other foods.

ADDITIVES AND PRESERVATIVES

We eat over a quarter of an ounce (10g) of additives and preservatives every day which amounts to over 8 lbs (3.8 kg) each year. My own common sense makes me realise that this continual cocktail of chemicals must be doing harm to some people. I am particularly worried about children, because children's systems retain a greater proportion of any given toxin, simply because their gastrointestinal tract is more easily penetrated. Children are also, of course, much more susceptible to carcinogens than adults are simply because babyhood and childhood are periods of rapid cell division.

My solution to this worrying scenario? Become a vegan or cut right down on meat, eggs and dairy produce and fish, and go organic as far as you can. This is particularly important as far as the youngest children in your family are concerned because they are the most at risk from the long-term health effects of additives, preservatives and pesticides.

● CAFFEINE ●

Many animal studies have shown that caffeine is a teratogen, that is a substance that causes physical defects in growing embryos. Caffeine has also been proved to accelerate the risk of infertility, miscarriages and premature births. This is particularly true during the first sixty days of pregnancy. Remember caffeine is also present in all Cola drinks, tea, chocolate, many over-the-counter drugs and any product where it is used for flavouring such as coffee ice-cream. Besides this coffee can cause palpitations, high blood pressure and raised cholesterol levels as well as increased acid secretions in the stomach. It can also aggravate fibrositic breast disease. Insomnia, anxiety, panic attacks and depression can be exacebated by caffeine.

While one cup a day of organic freshly brewed coffee as a treat is certainly not going to do you any harm, I would advise that you don't go much beyond this. However, the good news is that there are some excellent alternatives on the market including grain coffees made from cereals and fruits, chicory and dandelion coffee. Dandelion coffee brewed as a decoction from roasted ground dandelion root which is available from medical herbalists and other herb suppliers has the added bonus of being wonderfully cleansing and strengthening for the liver as well as purifying the blood. Do not mix it with milk or even soya milk because it makes it taste decidedly odd. Try and drink it black and unsweetened because the bitterness is what activates the liver, but if you can't manage it add a touch of honey or maple syrup. Half an ounce (15 g) of the root should be boiled for twenty minutes in a pint (600 ml) of pure water and then thoroughly strained before drinking. It can be reheated as needed.

Incidentally if you drink more than five breakfast-sized cups of coffee a day it means that you are clinically addicted to the caffeine in it.

I have stressed the importance of excellent nutrition well before conception and the reasons for it. During the latter half of pregnancy the foetus is, however, extremely protected by the placenta which can extract and concentrate vitamins from the mother's bloodstream for the benefit of the foetus. So the mother can suffer from an obvious deficiency without the foetus actually being affected at all. The growth of the foetus during the last half of pregnancy increases demands on the mother which the placenta ensures are met except in cases of extreme malnutrition. So if the mother's diet is inadequate during the latter half of pregnancy it is primarily *her* health that suffers.

PART TWO:
PREGNANCY

——

CHAPTER 4:

PREGNANCY

Preconceptal Care

• PREPARING FOR PREGNANCY EMOTIONALLY •

There are an awful lot of myths, both good and bad, attached to the role of mothering. Women are still reared to believe that it is the most fulfilling role they can have, but just as with anything else – like a job, a friendship or a marriage – there are days when being somebody's mother feels brilliant and days when it feels like a catastrophe. The responsibility can be both awesome and claustrophobic. One of my patients likened it to dragging around a heavy suitcase that she could never let out of her sight. And because she hadn't expected it to feel this way she felt terribly disappointed.

The hard truth is, whether a woman combines motherhood with a career, or makes it a career in itself, the role is an enormous commitment, a huge responsibility and just plain hard work. Our culture does not emphasise this but instead paints mothering as an easy, natural way to fulfilment. This primes many women for disillusionment. When the rosy picture painted fails to come true it doesn't occur to a self-doubting mother that the romanticised image is at fault, not her, and she saddles herself with a sense of failure.

Whether she is conscious of it or not, a good part of a mother's identity is linked to how well she feels she performs within her family. Mothering presents a primary area where she feels she is demonstrating her value. With some mothers the belief that she can never be good enough drags heavily at her self-esteem. For many the strain is very great. I interviewed a large number of my patients who were mothers for this book, and asked then how they felt emotionally about their mothering roles.

The first thing that shone through most clearly was what unequivocally hard work it is. But what also emerged with equal urgency was the lasting joy and sense of accomplishment it gave them. So be aware that some of your fantasies will come true and some of them won't.

• PREPARING FOR CONCEPTION PHYSICALLY •

We pass on our genetic blueprints to our children and sadly they tend to get scruffier as they go down the line. If your child suffers allergies, eczema, asthma or hay fever, if she has to wear glasses or has a mouth full of fillings, in spite of your best efforts at a reasonable diet, the chances are that you, your parents and even your grandparents were lacking in adequate nutrition exacerbating this problem generation after generation. I have some good news for you. You can change the pattern by looking after your own state of health **well before** you conceive. One of my greatest joys is to work preconceptually with women for at least six months to prepare for a really healthy conception. In my consulting room I have a wall full of pictures of the healthy babies born to women and men who were deemed by the medical profession to be infertile and of conscientious parents who wanted to give their child the best possible start in life. Looking at these pictures is a great source of joy for me, as it confirms that this is tangible proof of a really positive way to change the world with a healthier generation.

• PRECONCEPTUAL CLEANSING •

This is the ideal time to address an unhealthy lifestyle which may involve a junk-food diet, smoking, excessive drinking, drugs (both recreational and prescribed), weight problems or lack of exercise as well as high stress levels. It is advisable not to become pregnant until you have been off the Pill for at least six months.

I have covered the advantages and disadvantages of all sorts of contraceptive aids in one of my previous books, *Holistic Woman's Herbal*, (see Bibliography) and I have come down on the side of barrier contraception, including the condom, the diaphragm or even natural family planning. To me it seems a small price to pay compared to the pain and difficulty associated with anything else that medicine has so far come up with. Post-Pill amenorrhoea is common and I have worked with many cases of PID which, no matter how co-operative and conscientious the patient is, always proves uncommonly difficult to treat and requires a lot of hard work on the patient's part.

Once you have decided to try to conceive, short regular fasts of between 3 and 5 days of either fruit or vegetable juices, preferably organic and freshly pressed, coupled with a diet in between which is as near to vegan as you can get it is recommended. If you continue to eat flesh products ensure that they are organic as far as possible.

Men should give up smoking and drinking in order to improve both the quality and quantity of sperm. It has been shown that if a father eats a diet rich in Vitamin E for many months before conception this can have beneficial affects on the development of the baby's brain. In the Middle East foods which are rich in Vitamin E including sunflower seeds, sesame seeds, almonds and pine kernels are eaten daily to increase a man's physical strength and honey, pomegranates and olives are added to the list for the same reason. In Turkey I have seen salep, a gruel made from pounding up the roots of orchids given to increase a man's sexual stamina. It is not as horrid as it sounds because it is served liberally spiced and warmed in milk.

Some authorities recommend adhering to the marital requirements in the Old Testament which forbids sexual intercourse during menstruation and for a week afterwards. The argument goes that this regime encourages intercourse at times of highest female fertility and builds up a man's sperm count so that there is a better chance of fertilisation. It also increases the health of the prospective mother by giving her gynaecological organs a chance to regulate themselves during her cycle.

• HERBS •

There are many herbs which are specific for toning and strengthening the whole female reproductive system and they do so by feeding and nourishing these organs while toning, balancing and restoring vitality. They are safe to use over long periods of time and have very few side effects. My favourites are black cohosh root, dong quai root, liquorice root, squawvine, nettles and chaste berry. They should be taken in their tea form with the exception of black cohosh which needs to be taken in tincture form. The dose of black cohosh is 15 drops three times a day, and of the teas, one cup morning and evening.

Male energy tonic

2 parts: Siberian ginseng root   damiana
Korean ginseng root   saw palmetto berry oat seed
1 part: sarsaparillas   cardamom seed

This can be made as a tincture. In each case the dosage is a cup with every meal.

To ensure prostate health make sure the bowel and lymphatic systems are clean – consider asking an iridologist for advice. In addition take Bioforce's Prostasan in tincture form, fifteen drops three times a day before meals. Pumpkin seeds are rich in a male androgen hormone which will help to cleanse the prostate gland. Eat a couple of ounces (60 g) every day.

Female energy tonic

Equal parts of:
Siberian ginseng   sarsaparilla
dong quai   wild yam
agnus castus   ginger

25 drops three times daily.

• SITZ BATHS •

Sitz baths are an unbeatable and extremely effective therapy for restoring the health and vitality of the reproductive system, whether it be for men or women. I advise their use daily pre-conception, and twice daily if fasting. They work by drawing fresh blood into the pelvic area using hydrotherapy – alternative applications of hot and cold water dilate and constrict the blood vessels in the pelvic area. As the blood vessels dilate it encourages fresh blood into the area, and as they constrict the blood is forced away, thus encouraging a pumping action which concentrates energy in the pelvis and helps to remove stagnation and blocked energy.

Creating a sitz bath is easy, it simply requires a little organisation. You need two large plastic basins, big enough to sit in without getting wedged in them (a baby's plastic bath is ideal). Put four inches (10 cm) of the hottest water you can manage (without being ridiculous and scalding yourself) into one basin and four inches (10 cm) of icy cold water (you can even add a few extra ice cubes to keep it really cold) in the other. Place the two basins side by side and sit in the hot one while putting your feet in the cold one for three minutes allowing your legs to drop open so that you can splash hot water over your groin and abdomen. Then reverse the process. You will find that initially it will feel quite shocking. You may only be able to sit in the icy cold water with your feet in the hot for a whole minute, but gradually your stamina will build up to three minutes, then get out and vigorously dry yourself with a rough towel.

• EXERCISE •

Women need to concentrate on exercises that strengthen the muscles of the pelvic floor as well as some form of aerobic exercise that they enjoy. Over exercising may result in amenorrhoea which would be counter productive so take it steadily. Forty minutes of vigorous aerobic exercise three times a week is perfectly adequate. Men need to follow the same advice as chronic oxygen starvation from a stressful lifestyle degrades every other aspect of your life. Now, I know the next bit is a tall order, but you should be exercising in the purest, cleanest air you can find. Pure, unpolluted air is an absolute basic prerequisite for the health of everyone.

• SUNLIGHT •

Aim to get some natural light in your eyes and on whatever part of your skin is exposed for twenty minutes every day if possible. Natural light helps to protect us from infected organisms in the air, the skin and within our own bodies. It raises the number of white cells in the blood, increases the ability to deal with infection and interestingly natural fabrics are better transmitters of ultra-violet than synthetics. The heavier the fabric and the stronger the dye the more it filters out ultra-violet light. A recent report issued by Dr Galad and Dr Gorham on behalf of the American

Association for the Advancement of Science categorically stated, 'Vitamin D which is produced in the body when it is exposed to sunlight . . . protects against breast and colon cancer.' Men who work on submarines for months at a time are found to be not only more predisposed to dental caries but less fertile than those who get regular bouts of natural light.

According to the work of John Ott, a photobiologist who did an enormous amount of work in the area of sunlight and health, 20 minutes in a shaded area in the sun at midday, that is beneath a tree or under a porch, is perfectly acceptable.

• SKIN BRUSHING •

Get into the healthy habit of skin brushing every day and once you become pregnant continue on a daily basis. You will need to be more gentle during the last trimester over the abdominal area. Skin brushing is one of the simplest naturopathic techniques and I regularly introduce my patients to it with wonderful results. It exfoliates dead layers of skin and other impurities keeping the pores open and active, stimulates the glandular lymphatic and circulatory systems, rejuvenates the nervous system by stimulating nerve endings in the skin, and it revitalises and increases elimination. Remember that the skin is your largest eliminative organ and throws out one third of all your bodily impurities. If your skin is not eliminating and working well for you it burdens the rest of your eliminative organs with extra work. Besides this, the skin is capable of absorbing oxygen and exhaling carbon dioxide as well as absorbing specific nutrients that are rubbed on to it. The Russians for example have shown that minerals from sea water and sea air are absorbed through the skin and it is well known that Vitamin D is manufactured in the skin from sunlight. Skin brushing also helps with the distribution of cellulite leading to better muscle tone. It protects you from infection and many of my patients swear it prevents premature ageing. I can certainly promise it makes you feel wonderful, particularly when followed by hot and then cold showers for fifteen minutes afterwards.

The benefits of skin brushing must be tried and tested to be believed. You will feel clean, refreshed and much more alert. All in all, ready to cope with anything!

Because our skin is the largest two-way eliminative organ in our bodies – flushing outward by way of perspiration, and absorbing inwardly nutrients and vitamins from natural sunshine – it is worth taking special care of. The skin also breathes and absorbs oxygen while exhaling carbon-dioxide formed in tissues. The hundreds and thousands of sweat glands regulate body temperature and act as miniature detoxifying organs working to cleanse the blood and free the system suffocating poisons – they *should* operate to expel at least a pound of waste products daily.

Skin brushing stimulates the circulation helping to pump the blood down through veins and up through the arteries, feeding those organs of the body which lie near the surface. It also stimulates the lymph and adrenal glands, and has a powerful rejuvenating effect on the nervous system because of the hundreds of nerve endings in the skin.

By vigorous skin brushing over the major lymph glands, which are dumping stations for waste fluids, you can stimulate the expulsion of mucoid lymphatic material or impacted lymph. This is more commonly known as 'cellulite' and is the curse of many women. These lymph glands are situated behind the elbows and knees, under the arms, either side of the throat and especially in the groin. Skin brushing removes dead skin layers and other impurities, thereafter keeping the pores open and unclogged and increases the elimination capacity of the skin. It is important to remember that your skin brush is exclusively *yours*, not to be lent or borrowed by others. Used in conjunction with hot/cold showers it will help to stop colds.

Five minutes of energetic skin brushing is equivalent to twenty minutes jogging, as far as physical tone is concerned. It will build up healthy muscle tone and stimulate better distribution of fat deposits. All in all it can help you feel younger and gives a terrific sense of well being.

You will need a natural bristle brush with a detachable long wooden handle. The bristles will be quite stiff to begin with but will soften with use, so start with a light pressure and increase it. Your skin should be nicely pink and glowing.

Do not brush on the face – a softer and smaller brush is needed for that area. Nylon and synthetic fibres **won't do**. They will create static in the body and you would need to scrub for 20–30 minutes with a loofah or hand mitt to achieve the same effect as just 5 minutes brushing.

As your skin brushing is done dry brush on dry skin, it is important to maintain the brush properly. Wash it out once a week in warm soapy water, using natural soap. Rinse it well and dry in the airing cupboard thoroughly.

HOW TO SKIN BRUSH

- Using a natural bristle brush, start with the soles of your feet and a dry body. Brush upwards towards the heart from below and downwards from above.
- Brush vigorously up the legs and over thighs, remembering to brush towards the groin where the lymph glands are. Use a circular clockwise movement over the abdomen, following the line of the colon and do this about ten times. Avoid the genital area and the nipples.
- Brush palms and back of hands, up the arms to the shoulders but downward strokes on neck, throat and over the chest. To stimulate the important lymph glands under the arms, you use your hands to create a pumping action. Lodge the thumb under the clavicle bone and with all the fingers grip the pectoral muscle making sure the finger tips get right into the armpit. Squeeze and then release this area about fifteen times on each side.
- Use the handle on the brush to brush across the top of the shoulders and upper back, then up over the buttocks and lower back.
- This should take you about five minutes daily and first thing in the morning is the best time. Should you need to brush twice a day don't

brush too close to bedtime or you will not sleep. Brush every day for three months, then reduce it to two or three times weekly, changing the days each week.

- The scalp can be brushed to stimulate hair growth and free it from dandruff or impurities, or you may prefer to massage scalp with fingertips to move the scalp skin.
- It is fine for pregnant women to brush gently over their abdomen and is very helpful for circulation.

Never brush skin that is irritated, damaged or infected, or over bad varicose veins.

SHOWERING

After your 5 minutes skin brushing, it is time to remove dead skin cells by showering. Take a hot shower or bath for 2 to 3 minutes, followed by a cold shower for 20 seconds and repeat, moving the shower head from the feet upwards and then finish by holding it over the medulla oblongata at the back of the skull, letting cold water run down the spine. This method of hydrotherapy will alkalise the blood, clean the head and give a special boost to the glandular system and vital functions of the body.

• DENTAL AMALGAMS •

Twelve thousand published papers on the dangers of amalgams have so far failed to alter the opinion of the majority of the dental profession in this country as to its toxicity. However in Sweden because mercury fillings in pregnant women are acknowledged to affect the foetus, pregnant women are no longer allowed to have such fillings. On 14–17 June 1989 the University of Calgary Medical School presented the Canadian Federation of Biological Societies with a paper that showed that amalgam fillings placed in the molar teeth of five pregnant sheep produced mercury in foetal blood and amniotic fluid within three days of being inserted. Sixteen days later the mercury was evident in the pituitary glands, liver, kidney and part of the placenta and by thirty-three days (which is round about the time of birth for a sheep) nearly all foetal tissue had higher levels of mercury than the mother's did. During lactation the mothers had eight times as much mercury in the milk than in their own blood serum. Our own policy in the UK seems to be to actively encourage women to have dental work during their pregnancy.

By no means everyone reacts badly to mercury fillings but these should be properly tested by someone qualified and experienced in this field (see Resources Directory). Having said that I cannot emphasise how important it is to get the fillings removed in the right sequence by a dentist who is both experienced and fully qualified to do so. Any dentist simply won't do. Both Levenson and Huggins, the British and American leaders in this field respectively insist that the most negatively charged fillings be taken out first. Those who find they are mercury toxic and rush off to their dentists to have their amalgam fillings replaced willy nilly often get sicker because the protocol has not been observed and they suffer from an onslaught of mercury vapours.

If you are diagnosed as being highly sensitive to mercury (and tests done in advance can ascertain this) you should take 6 g of vitamin C mixed into water at the first signs of any adverse reactions. I have used the following programme very successfully over many years to detoxify mercury from the system.

1. Take a sauna or a Turkish bath once, or if you can manage it twice, per week as a lot of mercury is excreted through the skin.
2. Skin brush daily followed by a hot and then a cold shower.
3. Take three charcoal tablets three times a day with meals.
4. Take three tea spoons of spirulina daily in juice or two heaped tablespoons of Superfood (see Resources Directory).
5. Take six cloves of raw garlic a day. This is not as formidable as it sounds because four of these cloves can be buried in the following morning liver flush.

Liver Flush

On rising, thinly pare the yellow part of the skin of a lemon off a fresh lemon and slice the lemon. Put this in a liquidiser with four cloves of garlic, two tablespoons of olive oil, one inch of fresh ginger peeled and chopped and a large glass of any fresh juice of your choice. Liquidise it until it is creamy smooth and drink it slowly. The other two cloves can be used in salad dressing, garlic bread or part of the filling of a baked potato.

----

6. Two tablespoons of lecithin granules a day.
7. Six teaspoons of pectin powder in juice daily or three cups of cooked apple pureé daily.
8. Twenty drops three times a day of the following heavy metal detoxifying tincture:

6 parts of chaparral	*3 parts seaweed*
3 parts burdock root	*3 parts yellow dock*

Although mercury usually takes six months, and sometimes in poor excreters up to a year, to leave the body after all amalgams have been removed using this routine I have often succeeded in eliminating it from the tissues within twelve weeks.

A pregnant woman should never, under any circumstances, get her fillings removed while pregnant. Pregnant women can use the liver flush with impunity. It is ridiculous that in the UK pregnant women are actively encouraged to have dental work while pregnant or further amalgams are put into their mouths at one of their most vulnerable times. The detox programme is therefore only recommended for people who are having mercury taken out of their system while they are *not* pregnant.

• FINE TUNING •

The methods previously described are of necessity general, but if you are concerned or even merely curious that you may have a specific physical problem to address, I would suggest you seek the professional advise of an alternative practitioner who has good diagnostic skills. Many of the diagnostic methods your naturopath or medical herbalist use are ancient and well established and some are even beginning to be accepted by the scientific community.

Iridology coupled with Vega testing is my chosen diagnostic method. Iridology is the process used to diagnose conditions which involves analysing the iris of the eye. It reveals the presence of tissue inflammation in the body, its location and the stage it has reached. It is also a good indicator of constitutional strength, genetic patterns and inherent weaknesses. Vega testing concerns the ultra-fine measurements of cell-wall electrical activity from an acupuncture point on the hand or foot. Using a series of ampules containing anything from food to organ tissue, the practitioner can carry out a wide range of diagnostic tests, establishing whether a person has any intolerances to food, drugs or other materials. It can also detect the rate at which the body is affected by these and which organs are touched. It will also indicate vitamin deficiencies, tumours (and other cystic processes or infections), geopathic stress, psychic disorders, Yin Yang balance (body polarity), acid-alkaline balance and compatibility to a given medication. I am also trained in physical examination – although physical examination alone is far too inaccurate. Hair analysis, radiasthesia, tongue, pulse and ear diagnosis (which the Chinese have used for centuries), aura measuring and colour therapy come from the past and all show promise for future use. I have never felt the need to beg orthodox medics to recognise how valid my art is, both in philosophy and in practice. Alternative medicine is simply a direct continuation of the healing arts and understanding practised and developed for centuries.

Personally I always feel more confident if I go to a practitioner who is capable of conducting a good physical examination but who also has access to alternative means of diagnosis such as applied kinesiology, the aforementioned iridology and vega testing, mineral analysis done through hair tests, tongue and pulse diagnosis, and posture analysis. The time to begin addressing a specific health problem is only after you have found out what needs to be done and how it needs to be done. It saves a lot of time, worry and money. Please do not attempt to diagnose yourself. Even GPs may only be 50 per cent accurate with diagnosis without access to pathology laboratories and even there, their high-tech equipment is notoriously fallible as are its interpreters (see Appendix I). Too often allopathic practitioners are only concerned with a narrow bio-medical approach to the treatment of disease and this results in a fragmented treatment. That is besides the whole issue of it being poisonous.

The First Three Months

• SIGNS OF PREGNANCY •

Half of my pregnant patients know that they are pregnant without any chemical test to confirm it. They notice breast tenderness or enlargement, nausea, a decided lack of energy, more frequent urination, a subtle weight gain, and very commonly, great sensitivity to certain tastes or smells as well as a craving for specific foods and noticeable changes in appetite.

Less subjective signs include a missed period (not all women stop menstruating during pregnancy), a growing uterus which between the seventh and twelfth week of pregnancy will move from the size of a lemon to that of a grapefruit, as well as changes in the colour and texture of the cervix.

• SMOKING •

The single most important thing you can do to reduce risk to yourself and your baby is to stop smoking completely *before* you get pregnant or *during the first half* of the pregnancy. Not easy I know if you are addicted. Research on addiction indicates that nicotine works in almost the some way as heroin, cocaine and alcohol. In fact, recent research indicated that it may be even more addictive than both heroin and cocaine. When nicotine was administered intravenously to volunteers many of them could not tell the difference between the effects of nicotine and cocaine.

Women who smoke are more likely to reach the menopause early because of the toxic chemicals in the tobacco that affect the hormone-producing cells in their ovaries. They are more liable to osteoporosis, have a much higher risk of cancer of the cervix or the uterus, are less fertile and may have more difficulty with their pregnancies. They have more spontaneous abortions, still births and premature deliveries and their babies are smaller and at much higher risk than the babies of non smokers. So damaging is smoking considered during pregnancy that many midwifes will not even accept home birth clients who smoke during pregnancy. This is because nicotine constricts blood vessels, stemming the flow of blood through the placenta and so retarding growth. Specifically, the carbon monoxide and thiocynat in cigarette smoking reduces the baby's growth. Women who smoke have a higher risk of haemorrhage from the placenta. When a jolt of nicotine reaches the baby through the placenta directly, it will react by releasing epinephrine from its adrenal glands raising blood pressure, contracting blood vessels and diminishing the flow of blood to peripheral blood vessels and limbs. An alarming number of babies and children have cardiac defects and high blood pressure and these are believed to be transmitted by mothers who smoke during pregnancy.

Unsurprisingly, a woman who smokes will be depriving her baby directly in utero of oxygen by 30 per cent. This is a disastrous, life-threatening and suffocating situation for the baby because on the one hand nicotine stimulates the heart action and increases oxygen demand while on the other the carbon monoxide, one of the many deadly gases in cigarette smoke, cuts down any available oxygen to the minimum.

Cigarette smoke is also laden with polycyclic hydrocarbons, chemical substances that cause cancer. These are capable of entering the foetal bloodstream and causing cancer in the unborn baby which may not be diagnosable until early childhood.

Smoking during breast-feeding is equally unwise as the nicotine from smokers can be detected in the breast milk of nursing mothers. There is now a growing deluge of scientific literature showing that passive smoking produces more catarrh, coughs, ear infections and colds in the children of smokers and their colds are often more complicated, with bronchitis or asthma. So is their resistance to diseases such as meningitis.

• ELECTROMAGNETIC POLLUTION AND VDUS •

Of course we now live in an electronic age, but a growing number of studies all over the world are beginning to conclude that its side effects are killing us.

Electric and magnetic fields surround all electrical conductors whether they be giant power lines or the wiring in your house and electrical appliances. EMFs are made up of electrical fields and magnetic fields. Electrical fields are measured by voltage ranging from 240 volts domestically up to 400,000 volts on main power lines. The fields they create are rather like the static electricity you might feel when you get a small shock from a new carpet. Unless you live close to a major power line this isn't a problem because they can be shielded by walls and trees. But magnetic fields which are generated by electrical current wherever electricity is used can travel right through walls and cannot be shielded but only modified by the careful design of wiring and electrical equipment. There is also a growing concern about microwaves, television masts and transmitter – satellite dishes. In fact Solihull Council in the West Midlands has banned them in schools and within 37 feet (100 metres) of Council housing. Most transmission could be more safely sent by cable or fibre optics.

There is currently a tremendous argument as to whether EMFs pose an even higher risk to health than microwaves and the powerful vested interests of the electricity companies, computer manufacturers, electrical goods manufacturers and employers of VDU operators would have us believe there is not a problem at all. But you would be unwise to ignore the epidemiological studies that come from all over the world suggesting that we do have a major problem. EMFs have been linked to depression, heart attack, suicide, adult cancers and childhood leukemia, as well as more minor problems such as headaches, insomnia and irritability. Another piece of research that particularly concerns women was one where the electro-magnetic fields generated by electric blankets and heated water beds was found to increase the likelihood of miscarriages among pregnant women.

PROTECTING YOURSELF

If you are pregnant avoid VDUs if possible. This is particularly important in the first trimester when the baby is at it's most vulnerable.

Take sensible measures but do try to keep a sense of proportion. Remember two factors: duration and distance. Viewing a television set from 12 feet (3.6 metres) away will considerably reduce the effects of ELFs but sleeping on an electrical blanket which is switched on all night produces unacceptably high levels of ELFs. Microwave ovens and conventional electrical cookers generate large ELFs because of the heavy current they consume. If you can, and you have no respiratory difficulties, cook with gas. The Russians have, for many years now, banned the construction of buildings within a kilometre of power lines. You may draw whatever conclusions from that you like, depending on which side you are on. My advice would be the same as Dr Samuel Milham's, who suggests that if you are considering buying a house near a power line, buy a different one.

• SUN BEDS •

Sun beds are bad for everyone but particularly bad for women in pregnancy. Dr John Hawk, dermatologist and head of the photobiology unit at St Thomas's hospital in London, recently carried out a trial of thirty volunteers who used sun beds. The study concluded that not only did they get a *poor quality tan* but that sun beds had a potentially serious effect on the body's immune system. T-lymphocytes in the blood and langerhans cells in the pancreas were greatly reduced in number after a course of twelve sun-bed treatments lasting for thirty minutes each. Dr Hawk hypothesised that this subtle sabotage of the immune system could leave people more susceptible to colds, other infections and even skin cancer. More importantly, the light from sun beds exacerbates hypoglycaemia and insulin dependency increases. Couple this with the fact that 3 to 5 per cent of all pregnant women develop gestational diabetes anyway during the second half of pregnancy and you could be exacerbating this problem if you use sun beds.

• X-RAYS •

It has long been known that X-rays are carcinogenic and most doctors and dentists are now well aware that pregnant women should not be X-rayed. They are conversant with the link between the exposure of foetuses to radiation and childhood cancer which is now well documented.

It is estimated that the X-rays given to about 25 per cent of all pregnant women during the 1950s and 60s may have caused between 5 and 10 per cent of all childhood cancers throughout America and the Western world. X-rays also cause 'major birth defects, including small head size, mental retardation, skeletal deformities and eye and heart defects'.

In spite of the overwhelming evidence against the use of X-rays, hospitals are often sloppy about checking whether a woman may be pregnant so it is really up to you to take care of yourself and speak up. Bear in mind that if you have been X-rayed during pregnancy your baby will remain at high risk because she would be three hundred times more sensitive than a fifty-five-year-old to induction of cancer by radiation. Five-year-old toddlers are about five times more likely to get radiation-induced cancer later in life than an adult given the same radiation dose at the age of thirty-five. In his brilliant book, *Male Practice*, Dr Robert Mendelsohn believes that the evidence is overwhelming that women who have accumulated a lot of radiation during their lives have an increased risk of delivering a baby with Down's Syndrome and that it is this, rather than age alone, that is responsible for an older woman's increased risk. In addition, cancer research in America indicates that a significant percentage of women have inherited a gene, oncogegine AC, that is sensitive to X-ray exposure and that in these particular women even very brief periods of X-ray exposure could lead to the development of cancer.

If you are concerned about the damage X-rays may have done before you became pregnant take six tablets of kelp daily, which is a known protective against radiation, and 100 mg of co-enzyme Q_{10}, which researchers in Japan have found protects the body from harmful radiation. The sodium alginate found in all seaweeds acts as a chelating agent protecting the body from harmful affects of radiation by binding them with the radioactive elements and so enabling them to be excreted speedily from the body. Chaparral is also a well-known protective against radiation so take 15 drops three times a day in tincture form for two months.

Foods which help to protect against the harmful effects of radiation are apples, which are high in pectin and bind with radioactive particles, buckwheat which is high in rutin and protects against radiation, and also safflower, olives and avocado oils which supply essential fatty acids.

For more information on the pros and cons of allopathic testing during pregnancy see Appendix I.

• EXERCISE •

The Bedouin Arabs believe that to 'toil hard, walk far' is a certain recipe for ensuring healthy pregnancies and keeping their bodies in good condition. Certainly it is common for women in this culture to work hard amongst their crops and around their firesides almost right up to the hour of birth as well as continuing to ride horses and camels. Lack of exercise in pregnancy results in slack muscles, an excess of fluid in the body and often varicose veins. Although

I have often seen in books on pregnancy that women are advised not to undertake strenuous exercise such as sawing or chopping wood or riding horses, in my own experience I have found that my patients benefit extremely well from all sorts of vigorous exercise **provided they were used to doing this kind of exercise before they became pregnant**. Certainly women who acted as railway porters during the Second World War were renowned for having easy pregnancies and births.

My own feeling after long years of clinical practice is that oxygen is the most vital requirement for good health. Indeed I now refuse to treat smokers unless they are willing to give up smoking within a short time of consulting me. The only way you can bring more oxygen into your system is by deliberate exercise which is imperative for the correct functioning of all the organs in your body, but especially for the lymphatic system. I feel that vigorous exercise is probably the single most effective method of increasing both the well-being of the mother and the baby during pregnancy. Indeed it is even more important during pregnancy than at any other time since the body is placed under so many extra demands.

FLUSHBACK

When a pregnant woman exercises really vigorously, that is up to aerobic level, her blood is flushed upwards into her arms and legs away from her uterus. Of course this is true of any woman who takes exercise but once a pregnant woman rests afterwards the blood rushes back to the uterus and on to the placenta ensuring that its supplies are even more forceful than before the exercise was taken. Called flushback, this enables the foetus to amply make up for any lack of oxygen it might have experienced while the mother was exercising.

As I have stated earlier, a pregnant woman's blood volume increases by 40 per cent, and as the size of her heart increases her heart rate increases, the capacity of her lungs expands and the amount of blood pumped out by her heart also increases. All these changes in the body ensure even more oxygen-containing blood to the foetus and are very similar to the changes that take place when an athlete is training hard. A pregnant woman will also enjoy the same benefits an athlete experiences. That is, afterwards her blood pressure and pulse will go down which may be particularly helpful if she is predisposed to high blood pressure. It has also been found that the foetus is able to extract even more oxygen from the blood that it does get during the course of exercise.

CAN YOU EXERCISE TOO MUCH?

The following are symptoms you might experience if you overdo it: poor co-ordination (which may include tripping, stumbling or falling over, as well as poor judgement whilst driving), the feeling of extreme fatigue immediately after running, lowered resistance in general terms so that you easily catch infection and mild muscle soreness. Naturally, the last symptom will be common if you are just beginning to take up a new type of exercise. If in doubt the answer is to cut back on your exercise activity and see if you feel better. My general advice to pregnant patients is that they can do any type of exercise they like as long as it does not hurt and also that they are able to distinguish the normal aching of a muscle that is being exercised from the pain of injury.

Exercise that is normally conventionally recommended includes walking in good flat shoes, cycling, swimming and yoga. The latter is uniquely well suited to pregnancy because not only will it teach a woman good control with breathing and relaxation but it can help those who have difficulty sleeping. However, aerobic exercise does need to be part of a pregnant woman's routine and I have known women to do aerobic dance classes, horse riding, ballet dancing, cross country skiing, water skiing, tennis, badminton and other ball games as well as roller skating. In answer to the oft touted question, can exercising too vigorously or doing the wrong type of exercise harm the baby, the answer is that even strenuous exercise or a bad fall is very unlikely to do this. Indeed the mother is more likely to be injured than the foetus. Even while jogging while the mother may feel the impact of her feet hitting a hard surface, the foetus will be cushioned safely inside her amniotic fluid and the only problem is liable to be the uncomfortable bouncing of the womb or breasts at certain stages of pregnancy although there are specific support girdles available for this. The obvious exception to strenuous exercise is if premature labour or a miscarriage is threatened and in this case any strenuous exercise will bring on or exacerbate uterine contractions. Certainly our modern sedentary western lifestyle is not normal and my own experience is that while the extra load a pregnant woman carries with her may certainly slow her down, it should not preclude vigorous regular exercise. Remember pregnancy is not an illness. It is both natural and advisable to keep supple, active and strong during this time.

SLEEP AND RELAXATION DURING PREGNANCY

Rest and eventually sleep must follow exercise as night follows day, and so the cycle comes round again. It has often been said that the hours between twilight and midnight are twice as valuable as the hours from midnight to dawn as far as sleep is concerned and my feeling is that this must have some measure of truth in it when I observe the practices of religious orders that arise at three or four o'clock in the morning when they believe they are most mentally alert and go to bed when dusk comes.

It is very common to feel more tired than normal during the first few weeks of pregnancy but in general once entering the second trimester you will feel more energetic. The sensible rule to follow is to rest whenever you feel the need to and as your pregnancy advances try and make a habit of taking an afternoon siesta.

Be sensible and listen to what your body needs. Some stress is natural during pregnancy and controlled breathing, visualisation and meditation can be very useful. Sometimes unintentionally doctors, relatives, friends and acquaintances can be thoughtless and burden you with horror stories about birth and pregnancy, rather than stressing the positive encouraging aspects. Stress and negativity are guaranteed to send your immune system plummeting so try to maintain a balanced attitude. Mental health is not simply desirable it is essential for healthy body functioning.

The name given to the current avalanche of research information coming out of studies of the mind/body relationship is psycho-neuroimmunology (PNI). Scientists are now discovering that everything is connected to everything else in the human body, which, of course holistic therapies have acknowledged for centuries! Attitudes, emotions and mental processes can overload the PNI circuits and damage the immune system, so the mental pictures you create, the way in which you talk to yourself, is crucially important.

Visualisation and affirmations stimulate the immune system and change depression, personal attitudes, personality traits and life patterns. Powerful tools indeed!

VISUALISATION

Try this simple exercise when you are feeling unhappy. First consider what it is you fear at that very moment and then make a deliberate effort to shift your attention to something you CAN control. Store an idea in your mind precisely for these situations, and it should be a memory of something that once gave you special pleasure, or an exciting project you are planning, any situation in which YOU ARE IN CONTROL. This is the key. Learn to control your mind and stop the negative destructive thoughts that keep surfacing dead in their tracks. Refuse to let them ruminate or simmer. Keep this positive mental stream flowing with clear, sharp, colourful imagery and positive affirmations and that way you will keep a good stream of body hormones and nerve messages flowing through your body.

Think of your physical body as an instrument through which the mind plays. A good analogy is to imagine your body as a radio with an antenna attached to it called the brain. The mind is like radio waves and these invisible vibrations activate the radio into making sounds. Without them the radio would not work. Static radio waves mess up the radio. As it activates the physical body the mind functions with free will. Each of us can choose our thoughts, attitudes, what we choose to study and discuss, where to focus our attention, who we have as friends and how we behave. If we visualise ourselves as sick, weak or depressed this image will imprint itself on our bodies and the radio will pick up all sorts of static, so sounds will become jumbled. The brain antenna will affect the glands and evoke immune system depression. If we see ourselves as glowing with self esteem and health then this is the image that will be imprinted on the body and will evoke immune system strength and healing.

The best time to do this is when you are in an altered state of consciousness, practising yoga for breathing or meditation, or when you are under hypnotherapy. Before you fall asleep each night and when you wake every morning concentrate on positive thoughts and affirmations, visualising clear images of what it is you want.

I truly believe that when you want something to happen and focus on it with absolute desire it will happen. Pure heartfelt desire which stems from the spirit possesses awesome electromagnetic energy.

Focus. It is sometimes easy to forget that there is a baby amidst all the sensation and activity with which we surround ourselves. The commitment to birth doesn't come from the head it comes from the heart.

• MEDITATION •

Meditation generally needs to be taught although I have known people enter a deeply meditative state while bathing, painting, making bread, listening to music, running or gardening. Couch potatoes slumped in front of the television are far from relaxed or meditative, their sympathetic nervous systems remain in full flood. True relaxation involves a profound shift in various physiological systems. The mind barely dribbles over, there is a deep surrendering to the body's muscular system and breathing is slow and regular. The difference between relaxation and meditation is the self-transforming experience felt by the experienced meditator, not the simple reduction of stress. Meditation is particularly powerful when coupled with visualisation.

In the past Japanese and Chinese women were encouraged to practice meditation daily and to communicate with their babies in utero by tuning into the consciousness of the unborn child and sending positive loving messages to that child. A blissful way of simply enjoying being with your baby!

• NAUSEA DURING PREGNANCY •

This is commonly known as morning sickness (see pages 14, 85, 94, 101, 105–6) and affects almost half of all pregnant women during the first trimester to some degree or another. Nor does it confine itself to the morning. In a very few unfortunate women they can experience it well beyond the first trimester making what should be a happy experience downright miserable.

It seems a plethora of factors contribute to morning sickness including hypoglycaemia, low levels of B-complex vitamins, fluctuating dietary needs and particularly a steep increase in the hormone chorionic gonadotrophin. I found the herb that is particularly useful here, because it both tones and feeds the liver as well as balancing hormone production, is wild yam root. One of my most successful formulations consists of two parts wild yam root, one part chaste berry and one part ginger root. Decoct it and sip a quarter of a cup of warm tea every two hours. You may need to keep this up for several days and because it is fairly strong-tasting you may want to sweeten it with a little maple syrup. Its effects may take some time to become apparent so be patient.

Because many people believe that an insufficiency of vitamin B_6 can exacerbate morning sickness I have found that potassium broth with added nutritional yeast is not only easy to swallow but very comforting. It also seems to lessen the morning sickness.

Potassium broth

- Fill a large pot with 25 per cent of cut potato peelings quarter of an inch thick (1½ cm), 25 per cent carrot peelings, 25 per cent chopped onions and garlic and 25 per cent celery and greens. Add hot peppers to taste.

- Cover vegetables with water and simmer on a very low heat for 1 to 2 hours.

- Strain and drink only the broth and put the vegetables on the compost.

- Make enough for two days and refrigerate any leftover broth. Then start a new broth.

- To every mug of potassium broth add two desertspoons of nutritional yeast. Drink as much as needed whenever it is needed.

Please use organic vegetables if possible. It is important to try to consume produce which is least likely to have come into contact with toxic insecticides or chemical fertilisers while on a cleansing and detoxification programme, especially if pregnant and lactating.

My pregnant patients have found that they can balance their low blood-sugar levels by having snacks of dry biscuits spread with a little nut butter available to them on their bedside tables. Others have preferred popcorn. Some of my patients have had difficulty producing hydrochloric acid during the first few weeks of pregnancy and in these cases I have found digestive enzymes from pineapple and papaya helpful, particularly if taken when eating meals high in protein. In this instance the rules of food combining need to be meticulously applied.

In rare cases where nothing seems to stay down, I have found miso soup mixed with slippery elm into a thin gruel helpful, as well as soothing and quite palatable. Miso soup can be bought ready made-up from health food stores or it can be reconstituted from its dried powder form sold in packets.

One of the simplest most delicious teas for morning sickness is ginger root tea, although it doesn't work on some people as well as the wild yam combination.

Ginger root tea

● Grate 1 oz (3 og) of fresh ginger root and cover it with one pint (600 ml) of water. Simmer at a very low heat for 10 minutes, then strain. Add honey and lemon to taste.

This is delicious served either warm or, in hot weather, ice cold. Ginger root tea also makes a very useful formula for travel sickness, both in children and adults.

● MAKING LOVE DURING PREGNANCY ●

Men and women's response to this is necessarily individual as it is throughout their sex lives. Rest assured it is virtually impossible to hurt the baby even with vigorous intercourse. The foetus is well protected by your bony pelvis and the amniotic fluid in which she is cushioned. I have known some people to be disconcerted when they can feel the baby moving, especially towards the end of pregnancy and the obvious caution here is to adopt positions that avoid undue pressure on the abdomen. Orgasms throughout pregnancy, however they are induced are absolutely fine. Indeed sexual intercourse as a means of bringing on an overdue baby, coupled with orgasm, is known to work successfully to stimulate contractions because the combined affects of oxytocin release and semen in the vagina which is rich in prostaglandins combine to work wonders. To be most effective, semen should form a pool around the cervix so use the missionary position and lie still for half an hour after your partner has ejaculated so that the semen can collect around the cervix. During this time your partner can caress your nipples which even in isolation can produce contractions if continued for 20 minutes or more at a time. Whilst breast or clitoral stimulation is not guaranteed to get labour going it certainly will ripen your cervix making it flexible, soft and thinner so that it dilates more easily when labour gets underway. Masturbation will produce contractions even more quickly than intercourse.

Intercourse should be stopped if your bag of waters has broken, if your mucus plug falls out (don't worry it will form again within a few days, it simply means your sexual activities have been too vigorous), if you have vaginal bleeding, itching or a discharge, or if you feel any pain at all in the vagina or abdomen stop. If you have a history of miscarriage you should avoid intercourse during the first trimester.

WEIGHT GAIN

The general practice of monitoring your weight throughout pregnancy is, in my opinion, worse than useless and causes far too much unnecessary worry. If you are very underweight to begin with there is a slight chance that the baby will not be well nourished and if you are extremely overweight you may have a greater chance of urinary infections or a blood clot during pregnancy. But I have known many healthy overweight women give birth to happy healthy babies. In general it is important that your weight gain supports not only the growth of the baby but also the growth of the uterus, placenta and, most importantly, the necessary increase in blood volume. Tom Brewer, a nutritional expert paediatrician, considers a 40/50 lb weight gain optimal and my worry would be if a woman actually started to lose weight during pregnancy. If you are overweight to begin with you may experience some prejudice about a home birth, but never try and remedy this by going on a crash diet which would be bad for you and your baby. Simply eat a healthy diet as already outlined and you will be fine.

WHEN WILL THE BABY COME?

Unfortunately, as yet, there is no reliable test that can determine exactly when a baby will be born. The normal length of a pregnancy is 280 days from the first day of the last period. The birth of a healthy baby has been recorded after being carried in utero for a full year and more than half the number of babies delivered arrive before their scheduled date. What I am greatly against is induction of labour and scheduled caesareans, unless there are rock solid medical reasons for doing so.

The second three months

During the first trimester your baby will have grown from the size of a pea to that of a potato. While this may not sound much it is the most critical time for her future development, because it is during this period that almost all her physical characteristics are determined. She will also be at her most sensitive to external toxic influences such as drugs, alcohol, tobacco and X-rays. It is during the first trimester that the brain is fully developed as well as the nervous system and the final number of brain cells may be significantly less if nutrition has been severely impaired.

During the second trimester, and hopefully by the fourteenth week, any signs of morning sickness will have abated, you will feel the first stirrings of the baby and your appetite will improve. Many women tell me they feel even better during this period of a pregnancy than they did before they were pregnant.

● AFFIRMATION AND VISUALISATION ●

To those who have trouble relaxing and find it difficult to put on appropriate weight I suggest they visualise themselves beautifully round and full during pregnancy. Your emotions and feelings are crucial to your level of well-being and I have noticed that those women who really want to become pregnant and are full of joy and gratitude at being so, have far fewer complications during labour and delivery than women who are not consciously enthusiastic about their pregnancy. The same of course applies to a partner. This is not as odd as it sounds because it has now been suggested that it is during the second trimester a foetus is able to convert sensations into emotions and accurately tunes into the purely emotional content of his mother's and even his father's messages. Bonding begins to take place well before birth during this trimester but it is not automatic. It has been demonstrated that if a mother shuts down emotionally during pregnancy, for example, for whatever reason, the baby cannot bond unassisted and is at a loss. Strong intra-uterine bonding at this stage with your baby is her ultimate protection against the outside world's dangers and uncertainties and to a surprisingly large extent this bonding will determine the future of your relationship with your baby once born. So it is crucial that all the thoughts you have about your pregnancy and the impending birth, particularly from the second trimester on are as happy, comfortable and positive as you can make them. If this makes you worry that from now on you have to be perfect in thought, word and deed, as does your partner, please don't worry. Occasional negative emotions or stressful events are not going to affect your intra-uterine bonding adversely. Your unborn baby is much too resilient to be put off by a few setbacks. Problems arise only when she feels absolutely shut off from you, her mother, or when her physical and psychological needs are consistently and persistently ignored. Using the term we rather than I (after all you are now in a dual partnership) when doing affirmations is both realistic and important.

• YOUR WEIGHT •

If you are very fat you are much more likely to suffer from hypertension and to develop pregnancy diabetes, urinary infections or blood clots but I have known many healthy overweight women give birth to perfectly happy healthy babies and the height of the fundus (top of the uterus) is a much more accurate gauge of your baby's growth than constant weighing. Dieting during pregnancy will harm both you and your baby. Just aim to eat a really healthy diet cutting out all junk food, particularly saturated fat and sugar. It is underweight women who have more worries because there is a chance that the baby will not be well nourished, if they continue not to gain weight, particularly during this trimester. So please ensure your diet is optimal and if you are not inclined to eat make plenty of fruit smoothies with lots of superfood stirred into them. Not only do these taste lovely but they are very easy to absorb and digest.

• PREPARING THE BREASTS •

The second trimester is a good time to begin to minimise the chances of sore, cracked or bleeding nipples by exposing them to the sun on a regular basis and by massaging them with the following oil. Please note that provided the breasts are exposed by an open window you do not need to stand right up to the window's edge and can be half-way into the room. The natural sunlight will stream in and this will still help.

Breast and belly oil

4 oz (120 g) coconut butter   50 drops lavender oil (optional)
1 oz (30 g) almond or olive oil   25 drops neroli oil (optional)
3 teaspoons grated bees wax
(I use vitamin E oil)

Melt all the ingredients together in a double boiler and begin to massage your legs, belly and breasts at least once daily with this glorious smelling mixture.

Skin brushing the breasts is also particularly helpful and gently rubbing the nipples with a fairly rough flannel will stimulate them into becoming more erect and so easier for the baby to latch on to. Inverted nipples can be encouraged outwards by wearing a breast shield during the last few weeks of pregnancy. It is during the second trimester that you may notice some colostrum, a yellowish white secretion coming out of the nipples. You might want to contact the La Leche League International at this time (see Resources Directory). They are a self-help orientated group of women interested in promoting breast-feeding and many of my patients have spoken about the organisation glowingly. It also helps to talk with other women who have breast-fed their babies.

• EXERCISE •

Especially now that problems of morning sickness are beginning to fade, you should start getting into an exercise routine with some enthusiasm. Kegal or pelvic floor exercises are particularly important. Dianne Bjarnson, an extremely experienced lay midwife who has delivered many hundreds of babies in Utah, suggests that the relaxation between each contraction of a Kegel exercise is just as vital, if not more so, than the pulling up and tightening of the pubococcygeal muscles themselves. Her observation is that if the PC muscle is strengthened too tightly it actually has to rip in order to get a baby through, so a mother has to work not simply at tightening it but just as dedicatedly at relaxing the muscle. The relaxation between each lift should take at least as long as the lift and the holding. Done like this your birthing will be much easier.

• HOME BIRTH VERSUS HOSPITAL BIRTH •

Most women I talk to want a birthing in which they, not the medical profession, are in control. There are some who will accept induction, a forceps delivery, a planned caesarean, an epidural or other interventionist procedures, happy in the knowledge that their birthing is being managed by an obstetrician in whom they have confidence. While I am prepared to honour both points of view, the statistics I have studied clearly show that a home birth is much safer than a hospital one except in 5 per cent of high risk cases. I have noticed that women who are consulted about what they prefer and who clearly understand what options are available are much more likely to experience birthing as joyful and satisfying than those who are merely at the passive receiving end of care, even if that care is kind. Sheila Kitzinger in her excellent book, *Home Birth and Other Alternatives to Hospital* (see bibliography) has observed, 'When birth is disempowering, a woman feels degraded, abused and mutilated but when birth is empowering, the experience is enriching, her self-confidence is enhanced and she has a sense of triumph, **however difficult the labour was**.' The problem is home births, in the latter part of the twentieth century, are still regarded as abnormal since western governments have made a concerted effort to encourage women into hospitals for their births. Dr Robert Mendelsohn, Chairman of the Medical Licensing Committee for the State of Illinois, and a formidable paediatrician with more than twenty-five years experience, states in his excellent book, *Male Practice: How Doctors Manipulate Women* (see bibliography), 'An expectant mother should thank Providence for her good fortune if she has her baby in a taxi cab on the way to the hospital. The cab driver may not be much help, but at least he will spare her from all the purposeless, perilous and unpleasant intervention her obstetrician had planned to inflict on her. If the new mother has her wits about her she will ask the driver to wait, have the cord cut in the hospital emergency room, and then get back in the cab and take her baby home.'

Ideally, she should not have been in the cab in the first place because the safest place for a healthy mother to have her baby is not in a hospital, but at home.

Dr Mendelsohn insisted that his own daughters had their babies at home precisely *because* of the potentially dangerous technological wizardry that is available in hospitals to doctors. For example, electronic foetal monitoring immediately pushes the caesarean section rate up three times when it is first introduced and caesarean section is definitely riskier for women than vaginal births. Five times as many women die after a caesarean than after a vaginal birth and there is a much higher risk of infection and other problems. You are far more likely to have an episiotomy (a cut in the vagina to enlarge the canal) in hospital than at home or at a birth centre.

A planned home birth is, I believe, safer than a hospital one and care given by a midwife at home is safer than care from a midwife in hospital, and home birth with a midwife is safest of all. For those having their first babies both at home with a midwife it also safer than birth with an obstetrician.

If all this talk about home versus hospital births has piqued your interest, as I hope it has, I would recommend that you investigate Sheila Kitzinger's factual and well-documented book mentioned above. Also try and talk to some women who have had home births and armed with as many facts as possible make up your own mind. You will have other options available to you depending upon where you live. You may have the choice between an alternative birth centre linked with or perhaps completely separated from a hospital, a small GP unit in an independent midwife-staffed clinic which focuses on assisting and supporting physiological birth rather than obstetrics, or at home. Do feel free to explore your options, buoyed up by accurate information, then make a decision that feels right for you and for your family.

The third three months

By the time the foetus is entering its seventh month it is fully developed and during the last trimester makes heavy demands on nutrients, absorbing 84 per cent of all the calcium its mother ingests and 85 per cent of the iron. At this stage the baby will only weigh about a pound and a half and has a huge spurt in skeletal growth which is what all that calcium is needed for. The extra iron is needed for the baby and the placenta and to meet the demand created by the significant increase in maternal blood volume and in erythrocyte quantity. It is therefore particularly important that you get plenty of absorbable iron in your diet daily. Dianne Bjarnson particularly recommends blackstrap molasses. I like sprouted alfalfa and beet juice diluted half and half with other juices as well as spirulina. Of course the problem is that during this trimester you rapidly begin to feel like a beached whale and find that digesting food in any quantity is really difficult. Following the food combining rules is particularly important as is eating little and often. It is now that fruit smoothies really come into their own. Also the extra protein that you will need in this trimester is utilised twice as effectively if taken raw rather than cooked and sprouted seeds, grains, nuts, nut butters and nut milks are marvellous for this.

• EXERCISE •

If at this stage you feel too heavy to embark on your previous exercise programme at least try to go swimming or exercising in water and, when you bend down, squat rather than bend over. If you are not doing yoga at the very minimum sit on the floor in a tailor position or cross-legged with your back supported which will tone up the birthing muscles. To do this sit on the floor with the soles of your feet touching and your knees out and then press your knees towards the floor, not stretching too much but pulling and stretching the inner thigh muscles. This will tone up those muscles which sometimes become cramped during birth. The pelvic rock is also an excellent pre-natal exercise. With your hands placed directly beneath your shoulders and your knees beneath your thighs, arch your back up and then let it sag down slowly, not only can this help the baby's position but it relieves an aching back wonderfully. Also try this one. From a good straight standing position thrust your pelvis back so that your belly falls forward and your bottom sticks out and then return to the position you were originally in and repeat as needed. This helps to strengthen the muscles of the lower back, especially when in the last trimester there is a tendency to compensate for the weight of the growing bump by leaning back slightly in a sway-backed posture.

• LOVE-MAKING •

While some women prefer not to make love during pregnancy, especially in the last trimester because of their increased size and the extra effort or imagination it takes, I would recommend you keep up your sexual relationship with your partner for as long as you can. In this way he can be emotionally as close to your baby as possible. You are also less likely to drift past your expected date of birth because the prostaglandins in semen contribute to the ripening of the cervix which will assist you into labour. Try different positions. Pillows help. Rest several times during the day.

Pillows over which you can drape yourself while sleeping also help.

• PERINEAL MASSAGE •

This massage should begin six to eight weeks before the birth. This is particularly important for those women who have either been sexually or emotionally abused as children because, unsurprisingly, they develop a real tightness in the vaginal-perineal area. Dianne Bjarnson calls this a micro pelvis and believes it is the result of an unconscious shutdown of a woman's femininity denying circulation and therefore growth of the female organs. Dianne teaches all her patients or their partners to do the perineal massage, and although it takes time and effort it is a brilliant way of avoiding an episiotomy and so well worth it. Using olive oil or coconut butter and scrupulously clean fingers (if your partner is doing this he or she should wear a rubber glove) work a large amount of the cream in and around the vaginal area, the inner labia and the perineum. If you have a previous episiotomy scar make it the prime focus of attention. Work the cream into the area very thoroughly which may take four or five minutes. Then, using more cream as a lubricant, insert several fingers shallowly into the vagina and gently stretch the opening until you feel a very slight burning sensation. At this point maintain the stretch for several minutes or until the burning sensation stops. After only a few days, or at the most one week, you will find that there is a noticeable increase in flexibility and stretchiness. After a fortnight you may be able to insert the tips of five fingers before the burning sensation starts. Then after four weeks you will notice that you have worked the opening up to about 2½ inches (approx. 7 cm) which is about two thirds of the diameter of the average baby's head. At this point you can drop the massage off to every other day which will be enough to maintain the stretch and the softness. It is essential to continue to do your kegal exercises, remembering to relax your pelvic floor deeply and thoroughly in between each pull up. Prepared childbirth classes are highly recommended for learning control and relaxation. Let me say here that some women experience putting their fingers into their vagina as very painful to begin with or simply very physically difficult and this is where the help of a partner is invaluable. Dianne observes that in her experience few partners are prepared to do this but, if they are willing to assist babies emerge comfortably and easily. She has also noticed that for many women such intense attention to the vagina and perineum can bring up a tremendous amount of repressed emotion which, if properly handled, is no bad thing.

• NAUSEA •

It is not uncommon to experience nausea again in the last trimester and it is particularly important to deal with this quickly as at this stage both your and your baby's nutritional requirements are running very high. Catnip tea is particularly effective as it is high in vitamins, especially the B-complex ones. A couple of cups during the day and one just before bed will help.

• YOUR BABY'S MOVEMENTS •

Apart from the tests already mentioned that you can carry out yourself to check on your baby's well-being, you may notice that the baby becomes really active when you go to bed at night. Your natural reaction will be to change your sleeping position, which is the wisest response. The baby is signalling that she is uncomfortable and may be lying on the placenta or something else that is cutting off a little circulation so her activity will encourage you to turn into a different position enabling her to settle down. Do not in the last trimester lie on your back because it will cut off some of the baby's blood supply. Nor should you give birth lying on your back for the same reason.

CHAPTER 5:

A-Z OF MINOR AILMENTS DURING PREGNANCY

ANAEMIA

If a woman gets extremely breathless during pregnancy, midwives will often forget that this can be a sign of anaemia. An easy way to correct this is to take blackstrap molasses (providing you are not hypoglycaemic). Red raspberry leaf tea has a lot of natural iron in it which is easily assimilated into the system and, of course, encapsulated beet powder or freshly pressed beetroot juice diluted with other juices are all excellent sources of iron.

My feeling is that doctors often misdiagnose anaemia, especially during the second trimester when the blood volume increases sharply and the haemoglobin levels are naturally lower. Floradix (see Resources Directory) is a good source of iron. Symptoms of iron deficiency (apart from shortness of breath) include fatigue, weakness, palpitations and pale colouring. I do, however, point out to my pregnant patients that there are tremendous physiological and hormonal changes going on during pregnancy which could be the root of their need to rest and if this feels like the correct thing then please do it. Remember too, the advice on pages 47–8 about vitamin C assisting the absorption of iron.

ANXIETY ATTACKS

Again these may be caused by a lack of calcium and magnesium in the system, so the calcium tea will prove very helpful. Rescue Remedy will assist in dealing with the emotional content of the problem.

BACKACHE

This is caused by your burgeoning weight and the subsequent increased pressure on your body so remember to stand straight and tall and stick your chest out. It's very easy to end up with a sway back by compensating for your bump by leaning all your weight outwards with your stomach. Water beds are remarkably helpful as are good shoes such as Birkenstock sandals. If you decide to experiment with a water bed please make sure that it does not have electrical circuitry in it to heat it up. If you find the dimples on the back of your buttocks and then apply strong pressure with your thumbs, or preferably somebody else's thumbs, you can release the muscle tension in that area. A maternity girdle much like the abdominal binders worn by primitive tribes is also very helpful. The exercises on page 92 are good as is the following exercise. Bring knees up to the chest bent and hold them there for thirty seconds before lowering them again. Sitz baths can alleviate backache as of course can osteopathic and chiropractic treatment carried out on a regular basis by a practitioner who is experienced with pregnant women. Some of my patients have told me that wheatgrass juice has helped to remedy their backaches and any deep heat oil (see Resources Directory) massaged into the back is wonderfully soothing.

BLEEDING GUMS

Ensure that your vitamin C content is very high. Red raspberry leaf tea is helpful here. Also make sure you have your calcium tea every day. Use a soft toothbrush and massage your gum with your fingers after every brushing with tincture of propolis or myrrh.

BREATHLESSNESS AND PALPITATIONS

This is generally a sign of anaemia (see page 95).

CANDIDIASIS (THRUSH)

Candida Albicans is a common yeast that lives in the digestive tract of everyone but it is only when our immune system has become compromised by antibiotics, steroids, poor diet or prolonged stress, environmental chemicals or prolonged damp living conditions that the form of these changes to a fungal one. Pregnancy places an extra burden on the immune system so thrush can be quite common in women during this time. The problem is if the mother has it when she is giving birth, the baby can pick it up in her mouth as she comes down the vagina and you will notice white spots in her mouth and on her tongue that looks like milk curds but don't rub off. Sometimes her whole tongue will go white. Often I can smell candida albicans on women but its most common manifestation is a cottage cheese type of vaginal discharge, fungal infections growing beneath the breasts or in the mouth or intense anal itching. If you are getting a persistent uncomfortable vaginal discharge you *must* get it properly checked out by going to see your doctor who will take a swab and send it to a path lab. Other types of vaginal discharge are common in pregnancy and need to be treated accurately.

My treatment begins with a good wholefood vegan diet including at least 50 per cent raw foods. Practitioners who preclude yeast, as many do, puzzle me. The difference between food yeast and the candida organism is rather like the difference between a bay tree and a monkey puzzle tree. While I might advocate the exclusion of brewer's yeast and substitute an inactive nutritional yeast (see Resources Directory), I certainly do not exclude fruits and vegetables from the diet and I ask my pregnant patients to take plenty of organic olive oil and eat as much garlic as they can manage. I have found a very good way of eating garlic in huge quantities, is to slice up the raw cloves and eat them piece by piece with mouthfuls of fresh ripe pears. The liver flush (see page 76) which is high in garlic is a very pleasant drink. Olive oil actively discourages the growth of the fungus and so should be massaged liberally around the vulva and labia or anus. Apart from garlic there is a wide range of herbs that are extremely effective against fungus including black walnut, T-tree and horsetail. T-tree pessaries inserted vaginally are extremely helpful as is cervagyn cream (see Resources Directory). Herbs that assist to build the immune system include echinacea and pau d'arco. Bio-acidophilus will also help to replace the benign flora in the colon. Obviously don't wear tight pants which cut off air from the area and make sure all your underwear is cotton or go without underwear. Drying the area with the cold air from a hair dryer is very soothing before massaging with cream or olive oil. The items I would advise cutting out of the diet completely while you are infected include fruit juice which is too concentrated in sugar and any other sweetener such as honey, maple syrup and molasses as well as sugar, because sugar distresses the immune system. Fruit should be eaten fresh and whole or frozen (as in fruit smoothies, see page 35).

CONSTIPATION

It is extremely common for the whole body to slow down in the first trimester because a woman's energy moves down into her digestive tract, not unnaturally. The problem is constipation can be one of the causes of miscarriage. As a fully qualified colonic therapist I wouldn't hesitate to give colonic irrigation provided there is no history of miscarriage in the family or previously with the woman concerned. I have also found Dr Christopher's lower bowel tonic extremely helpful. I make a variation of it.

- -

Intestinal Corrective Formula No 1

The combination of herbs in this formulation cleanses the liver and gall bladder, starts the bile flowing and stimulates peristalsis so that the layers of encrusted ancient mucus in the colon can gradually slough off as the bowel is rebuilt, resulting in the better assimilation of food. It also helps to heal inflamed areas in the colon and relaxes tension. While it does contain small amounts of Golden seal I have removed this as it is an oxytoxic herb and replaced it with garlic and wild thyme, so the formulation is as follows:

1 part of barberry bark	*fennel*
cayenne pepper	*2 part cascara sadgrada*
lobelia	*½ part wild thyme*
red raspberry	*½ a part garlic*
turkey rhubarb	

Buy all these herbs in powdered form and mix them together by sieving them. Fill size 0 gelatine capsules with the mixture. Begin by taking two capsules three times a day with meals or if you don't eat three times a day, take two capsules with every meal that you do eat. The aim is to achieve a bowel movement for every meal ingested. If you get diarrhoea cut the dosage down. If you cannot get a bowel movement raise the dosage gently until you can. The dosage of this formulation produces very individual results and must be monitored and adjusted according to your own unique response.

- -

This formulation must of course be coupled with a good diet and exercise programme unless you are not eating at all because you are so nauseous in which case I would recommend that you see a colonic therapist (see Resources Directory).

If constipation is mild but still needs some help I would recommend Intestinal Corrective Formula No 3 liquidised into fruit smoothies. Designed by my teacher, Richard Schulze, it will draw out impacted faecal matter from the wall of the colon together with residual toxins including heavy metals and radioactive elements. The charcoal in the formulation draws out 2,000 different kinds of chemical drugs from the bowel and through the bowel wall from the blood and lymphatic system. While normally I wouldn't allow a woman to do any serious detoxification during the course of pregnancy, this formulation is so gentle and so safe that I am perfectly happy using it at any time during pregnancy. It goes down particularly well if it's mixed with fruit smoothies (see page 35).

Intestinal Corrective Formula No 3

2 parts psyllium seeds
ground flax seeds
powdered charcoal
1 part each of bentonite clay

fruit pectin
carob pod
slippery elm bark
liquorice root

Make sure all the ingredients are finely powdered and mix well. Take one heaped rounded teaspoon, two to five times daily in a fruit smoothy mixing in a blender. Drink an additional 16 fl 02 (450 ml) of any type of liquid after each dose of this formulation.

Linusit Gold, available in Health Food shops which is organically grown flax seed, can be used in isolation mixed into soups, cereals or soya yogurt for mild constipation.

COUGHS AND COLDS

For coughs and colds take a teaspoon of garlic or onion syrup every 15 minutes and massage the chest with olbas oil as well as taking 360 drops a day of echinacea tincture until the infection has passed. A delicious and very effective tea for a cold is ginger tea with honey and lemon, a generous pinch of cayenne pepper, and a crushed clove of garlic in each mug. Use hot mustard foot baths to decongest the head and a salt water douche into the nose using a nasal spray to open up and decongest the sinuses. If the throat is sore, spray neat echinacea tincture down it or gargle with it as often as needed.

A cold that is properly managed should last for only two days and should flow purposefully and freely. Think of it as a natural purification process. Any cold that is discouraged and suppressed with chemical remedies (which you should not be taking during pregnancy anyway) may drag on in one form or another for two or three months. The correct adage is, 'If you feed a cold you will have to starve a fever.' So while you shouldn't fast during pregnancy, I would advise you go on to vegetable broth and soupy grains with lots of onion and garlic in it for twenty-four hours to give your digestive system a rest together with lots of freshly pressed citrus fruits.

CRAMP

In pregnancy it is very common for lack of calcium to cause leg cramps so make sure you have your calcium tea (see pages 51, 102) every day. Lack of vitamin B can also cause leg cramps. If you get a cramp, flex your foot upwards towards your knee and get somebody to massage your legs every day from the thigh working down to the foot, provided you don't have varicose veins. Don't cross your legs. Some women find that support hose helps. Valerian root tea is a specific herb indicated for muscles and ligaments and excellent for relieving muscle cramps and backaches due to tired muscles. An alternative to valarian root tea is Ginkgo Biloba tincture, 10 drops every fifteen minutes until the spasm is relieved internally. Massaging the legs with deep heat oil (see Resources Directory) will also relax tight muscles amazingly fast. If you get what some women call 'spider legs', that horrid creepy crawly feeling under the skin, it may be due not just to lack of calcium but lack of potassium in which case the potassium broth is indicated (see page 86). Tramping up and down in a bath full of cold water may also prove helpful because it assists the circulation. This is also very useful to sooth varicose veins.

DIARRHOEA

It is common to get diarrhoea just before you go into labour and indeed is a sign of labour, but if you have diarrhoea at any other time try slippery elm gruel or the Intestinal Corrective Formula No. 3 (See page 99).

DIZZINESS

This is common in the first trimester because the muscles of the blood vessels relax from all the extra pregnancy hormones which means when you stand up there is more gravity to work against to enable the blood to reach the brain. Remember to change your position slowly so that your blood vessels have time to adjust and eat small meals rather than large ones, little and often. Dizziness coupled with high blood pressure and albumin in your urine is not normal so if you have any worries consult your doctor.

EARACHE

> *Your ears are very delicate and sensitive and can be damaged easily by inappropriate treatment, if in any doubt at all about the cause of an earache please consult your doctor.*

If the earache is merely the result of a chill put a few drops of mullein or garlic oil into both ears (even if only one ear is infected) and plug with cotton wool. A hot foot bath will ease the pain of earache as will any source of heat applied locally to the ear, for example lying on a hot water bottle that is well wrapped in a towel.

FATIGUE

Many of my pregnant patients tell me they feel overwhelmingly exhausted in the second month of pregnancy and this is often the result of poor nutrition. This is where the pregnancy tea and calcium tea, together with iron-rich foods, work very effectively (see pages 49, 50, 51, 100, 102, 117).

Energy tea

Equal parts of Siberian ginseng, liquorice root, prickly ash and yellow dock. Make this as a double-strength decoction by using one ounce of the herbs and simmering it in only half a pint of water. After 20 minutes turn off the heat and allow it to steep overnight and then take a tablespoon every hour throughout the day. Do not continue with this for longer than a few days. By that time it should have done the trick. If it hasn't, please consult a professional medical herbalist.

HAEMORRHOIDS (SEE PAGE 109)

HEADACHES (AS A RESULT OF TENSION)

A headache which is due to tension can be soothed by pacing a steaming hot wet towel around the back of the neck while putting your feet in a basin full of hot water. Alternatively, take a brisk walk making sure your hands, feet, head and neck are well covered and breathe deeply while you do so. On your return drink half a cup of the following soothing tea every half hour until the headache subsides:

2 parts camomile	1 part vervain
1 part vervain	½ part valarian
2 parts lemon balm	

In between cups of tea lie down in a darkened room with a pillow on your knees to ease any strain on your back and neck. Please note chronic headaches can be a result of liver congestion, poor circulation, constipation, hypoglycaemia, food intolerance, sinusitis, arthritis, spinal lesions, anaemia, the side effects of a lumbar puncture, meningitis, a brain tumour, high blood pressure and eye strain.

A severe headache with vomiting may be the result of intra-cerebral haemorrhage. Some headaches are serious and will need diligent investigation from your doctor so please do this before adopting self-medication with herbs.

HEARTBURN

To some woman during pregnancy this can be a real plague, particularly in the last trimester or if they are badly afflicted by morning sickness. The first and most important thing to remember is the food-combining rules (see page 00). The second is never to take any anti-antacids during pregnancy (see page 00). The third thing is to chew your food really really well, even swishing juices around the mouth to mix them with saliva before digestion, and not to drink anything with meals except for potassium broth or juices. Tea, coffee, cigarette smoke, all irritate the stomach and exacerbate heartburn. Meals should of course be small and frequent. Fresh papaya if you can get it or papaya tablets are very helpful because they are massively high in digestive enzymes. Mucilaginous herbs like slippery elm and marshmallow sooth the digestive tract. You can make a cup of slippery elm gruel easily by liquidising a heaped teaspoon of slippery elm powder in warm soya milk with a touch of honey and cinnamon. Mix equal parts of powdered peppermint, liquorice and fennel into a paste with water. This is quite tasty and you can eat it off the spoon. Take a heaped teaspoon before any meal. Alternatively you can make a tea of these herbs using the leaves and roots and sip it throughout the day.

HIGH BLOOD PRESSURE

Often this is simply the result of oedema which constricts the veins and in this instance the calcium tea can be very helpful. Cayenne pepper building up to one rounded teaspoon three times a day in water or juice will equalise both high and low blood pressure. Garlic and hawthornberry tea are also excellent tonics for high blood pressure and of course exercise and peace of mind can lower blood pressure dramatically. Extra sources of vitamin E may be helpful for those suffering from low blood pressure.

HYPOCALCAEMIA

Remember protein-induced hypercalciuria will occur steadily for hours as calcium floods out of the body through the urine, the result of eating a meat-containing concentrated protein like meat, fish or dairy products. A vegan diet, unburdened with heavy protein loads from meat, fish or dairy products, creates less calcium loss from the body. Dianne Bjarnson, who is not herself a vegan, feels that milk stops the absorption of just about everything in pregnancy and should be avoided while pregnant. She has a recipe for calcium tea as follows:

Calcium Tea

Take a heaped teaspoon of oatstraw and simmer it to break it down (oatstraw powdered and put in a capsule simply does not break down in the same way) and then having taken it off the heat, steep a teaspoon of comfrey and a teaspoon of horsetail into it. Dianne recommends three cups in the morning and feels it sets the system up for proper absorption of nutrition for the rest of the day.

Dianne has observed that women taking inorganic calcium supplements, even those that are biochelated, produce placenta which look just like a smoker's placenta, that is one that is coarse and gritty and cannot feed the baby properly. She notices that babies born attached to this kind of placenta tend to suffer from nasal drip and mucus coming up from the throat for several weeks after birth and she feels this is the result of inorganic calcium. She also recommends chewing almonds that have been left to soak overnight (the soaking allows the calcium into the system a lot quicker) and, like me, she is a great believer in freshly pressed carrot juice which is massively high in calcium. Her calcium tea is readily accepted by babies who are calcium deficient and if they don't like the taste, although most of them do, just add a little drop of molasses. Calcium deficiency in babies is often manifested as constant crying and fussiness. Hypocalcaemia needs to be watched for particularly after birth if a woman is suffering from gestational diabetes (see page 104).

HYPOGLYCAEMIA

During pregnancy any craving for sugar will usually get worse and the answer is not doughnuts or honey but plenty of fresh fruit and juice together with the following pancreas combination which should be taken throughout pregnancy. Not only will it build and strengthen your pancreas but it will ensure that your baby is born with a better chance than you of not having hypoglycaemia which is extremely widespread and often remains undiagnosed being labelled as merely emotional or psychological.

Throughout the pregnancy hypoglycaemics need to take high-quality protein including pulses and sprouted seeds as well as plenty of raw and cooked vegetables. A power-packed drink which is easily made consists of a handful of soaked almonds, a cup of water, a banana, some pineapple juice, two tablespoons of nutritional yeast and a handful of Linusit Gold blended at high speed until the seeds have thickened the drink. This is a great way of getting high vibration protein into the system.

Pancreas formulation

Equal parts of
finely powdered uva ursi   *mullein*
cayenne pepper   *oregano grape root*
cedar berries   *yellow dock.*
liquorice root

Take three capsules three times a day.

If this is coupled with the adrenal formulation on page 105 it works spectacularly well.

Women who suffer from gestational diabetes, that is they become diabetic during pregnancy, need to be very strict about their diet. They will often have larger babies which look a bit puffy. The calcium tea in the first few days of the baby's birth both for the mother and the baby is an excellent aid, particularly if the baby goes a bit limp after birth. The diabetisan formula from Bioforce (see Resources Directory) is also very helpful. Jerusalem artichokes are said to be very high in insulin and make a very pleasant soup. Add a little apple cider vinegar towards the end of the cooking to lessen the chances of you getting wind as Jerusalem artichokes are notorious for creating it.

INSOMNIA

The first and most important pre-requisite is daily exercise. If you do not exercise on a regular basis while pregnant the acetyl choline will build up to such an extent that your nervous system will become fogged making you irritable and jumpy. Aerobic exercise (and remember you can reach an aerobic level simply by walking briskly) is the *only* exercise that will burn this off. Exercise outdoors is better than inside and you will have noticed yourself how a day spent outdoors in a park or on a beach makes you feel very tired when you return home.

Skin brushing followed by alternative hot and cold showers especially on the head is a wonderful way to calm the nervous system down. It should not be done just before bed as it will keep you awake.

Surprisingly walking barefoot on soil or grass just before going to bed also helps. I know this sounds very odd, but what happens is that the excessive electrical charge built up in the body during the course of the day while walking on synthetic surfaces is released and literally grounded into the natural substance beneath your feet. Aim to walk barefoot on grass, sand or soil for five minutes a day. Dry your feet vigorously afterwards with a rough towel and then put on warm socks followed by shoes or slippers. Ideally this should be done just before bed. It will certainly give the neighbours something to think about!

Alternatively if you don't have a garden try going to bed in a pair of loose fitting wet cotton socks covered by a large pair of woollen socks. This sounds odd and uncomfortable but actually it isn't and it does induce sleep. Ensure that you sleep in natural clothing and 100 per cent cotton sheets. Before going to bed take a bath at 34 to 36°C (94 to 97°F) with 10 drops of camomile oil added to the bath water. This will help to reduce congestion of the brain and spinal cord. At night-time sleep with your window slightly ajar or, if safety precautions preclude this, have an ioniser plugged in by your bedside.

Experiments in America have proved that paradoxical intention is very helpful for chronic insomniacs. This means doing the opposite of what you want in order make it happen. For example, in one experiment insomniacs were asked to stay awake as long as possible and to note their thoughts. One woman reduced her wakeful periods from ninety minutes to five and a half minutes! This is a bit like Mary Poppins' technique singing a lullaby 'stay awake; don't go to sleep . . .'

Go to bed only when you are tired and once there do not watch the television. Indeed you should not have a television set in your bedroom because of the electromagnetic fields around it (see pages 79–80). Do not read or lie awake worrying. If you don't fall asleep quickly get up, go out of the bedroom and do something until you feel ready to try again. Eat lightly before going to bed. Set the alarm for the same time every morning including weekends. Several cups of valarian tea sweetened with honey may be helpful or you could try Valariana comp tablets taken at the same time each night. Take one and, if necessary, increase the dose to two. They are extremely effective (see Resources Directory).

But before resorting to these try every other non-herbal measure I have suggested first. Don't deny yourself lie downs and little naps in the day, particularly during the first few months of pregnancy and the last trimester when you do feel much more tired.

IRRITABLE BOWEL SYNDROME

A finely orchestrated combination of Intestinal Corrective Formulas Nos 1 and 3 can be extremely helpful for sustaining a woman through pregnancy who suffers from irritable bowel syndrome. Aloe vera juice (see Resources Directory) two tablespoons at a time in fruit juice as needed can be very soothing.

MORNING SICKNESS

If you come from a family that suffers from morning sickness it will be worth your while building up your adrenal glands before you get pregnant as adrenal exhaustion can certainly exacerbate this condition.

Adrenal tonic

The following formulation will help to restore hormonal function and support the adrenal glands while regulating blood sugar and increasing the body's resistance to disease thereby counteracting stress.

2 parts Siberian ginseng   *one part each of echinacea, wild oats, bladderwrack, gotu kola.*

Take 15 drops three times a day with meals in tincture form. Stay on this formulation for at least three months before conception.

Apart from following the advice on pages 85 and 94, raspberry leaf tea may also help if used little and often. A cup should be sipped every couple of hours. Dianne Bjarnson has found with her pregnant clients that apple cider vinegar in hot water with honey and, if you can handle it, a pinch of cayenne pepper works, mainly because she feels it helps to get the digestive system going. If morning sickness persists into the third trimester catnip tea helps. Morning sickness can be exacerbated by lack of B_6 as the increased stress in the body depletes vitamin B_6 quickly during pregnancy, particularly because it is water soluble. A pregnant friend of mine swore by popcorn rolled in nutritional yeast as the only food that she could get down during her first three months. Wrist bands sold in chemists for travel sickness are also very useful as is the good old-fashioned hot water bottle, together with bed rest, a good book and ginger tea (see page 87).

For women who are in extreme difficulty and cannot stop throwing up, I have used mineral enemas to balance their systems and assist with their rapid loss of electrolytes. I add two sachets of iron water (see Resources Directory) to two litres of purified water administering this warm. Women who have never had an enema before can initially feel very discomforted by the mere thought of the whole process but it provides such a relief that ultimately they are very grateful.

NOSE BLEEDS

If you can bear it, sniff a pinch of dry cayenne pepper up each nostril. If you can't, put ice cubes on the back of your neck.

MUSCLE PAINS

Some women get persistent shooting pains down their thighs in the last part of pregnancy but often this can happen earlier. These are caused by your baby pressing on specific nerves. Have someone else press the muscles inside the thighs and between the hip bones and the pelvic bones really firmly until the tightness disappears. This is also wonderful for the dreadful ache some women suffer throughout the crotch area and it cannot hurt either the mother or the baby.

OEDEMA

This occurs in the second and third trimesters and a very close eye needs to be kept on the diet to make sure that you are not tipping into pre-eclampsia. Pregnancy hormones encourage connective tissue in the body to swell and retain extra fluid which is there to protect both mother and baby but excessive fluid is a sign of stressed and overburdened kidneys. This can be the result of not only a physical imbalance but emotional stress. Herbal diuretics work safely and extremely well on water retention and should be taken at the rate of four or five cups a day. My favourites are dandelion leaves or root, cleavers, uva ursi and nettles. Alfalfa, while not a diuretic, is wonderful for cleansing the bloodstream, as is spirulina.

URINARY TRACT PROBLEMS

In pregnancy the tubes that carry the urine from the kidney to the bladder, the ureters, get dilated, especially the right one. This is the result of the pressure created by the expanding uterus. In addition, hormones cause the smooth muscles of the lower abdomen to relax. This loss of muscle tone can impede the flow of urine through the system, making bacterial infection much more likely. This is particularly true later in pregnancy. Pyelonephritis affects up to 10 per cent of pregnant women and symptoms include fever with chills and shaking beginning gradually but coming on fast and strong. There is also pain in the back just below the ribs and the right side may be more affected than the left. Sometimes there is pain in the abdomen and there may be frequent weeing and general discomfort. Pyelonephritis can cause premature labour and it needs immediate attention. Cystitis which is an infection in the bladder only causes a burning sensation when urinating and if not attended to can blossom into Pyelonephritis. Either of these conditions needs urgent attention either from a professional medical herbalist if you wish to be treated by herbs, or from your local GP. I immediately start my patients on unsweetened cranberry juice (you can buy frozen cranberries from supermarkets), a complete abstinence from sugar and half a cup every half hour of the following tea.

Tea for bladder infections

2 parts corn silk   1 part dandelion
2 parts buchu   1 part yarrow
1 part nettle

- Infuse the above.

Also take 360 drops of echinacea tincture over the course of twenty-four hours. I am perfectly happy treating both kidney and bladder infections providing they are caught early enough. Herbs work very well with them. I will also help relieve pain with hot ginger poultices applied to the kidneys and intensive bodywork both on the back and the soles of the feet.

VAGINAL BLEEDING

It is thought that up to 40 per cent of all pregnancies miscarry in the very early stages and are mistaken for heavy or late menstrual cycles. Excessive bleeding, cramping and clotting which are often associated with irregular or heavy menstrual cycles are sometimes simply spontaneous miscarriages. If this happens within the very early weeks of pregnancy low progesterone levels may be the cause. If this is the case I would normally put a woman on 1600 mg daily of Siberian ginseng powdered in capsules right through her pregnancy. Those who start to cramp later in their pregnancy over the course of the sixth or seventh month or even the eight month can take double this dose for a week or two and it will normally stop a miscarriage or premature birth. If in doubt as to whether a low progesterone level is the cause of your miscarriage your doctor can give you a test to determine if this is the case. Please note synthetic progesterone is **not** recommended as it may cause birth defects in children. An alternative progesterone-stimulating herb is wild yam root, but in my experience it is not as effective as Siberian ginseng.

Miscarriage can also be the result of too much stress, an inadequate diet, trauma, weak uterine muscles or a body that is too toxic to carry a baby full term. It is for this reason I place heavy emphasis on cleansing and detoxifying to enable infertile couples to conceive and women predisposed to miscarriage to carry to full term (see Appendix III). In many cases herbs can provide that extra nourishment and strength needed to correct the problem and it is **absolutely essential to go to bed and stay there resting completely until the crisis has passed**. That means don't even get out of bed to go to the toilet, use a bed pan. One of the worst things you can do is try to get back on to your feet and take control of your household again. This is a time for letting go and trusting others to do that work for you.

Of course in any trauma Rescue Remedy comes into its own both for the carers and patient. Use it liberally as often as needed.

VAGINAL DISCHARGES

The first and most important thing is to get the discharge properly analysed by your doctor. While it is common to get more vaginal discharge during pregnancy there is also a chance that it may be an infection other than thrush. If this is the case and you would prefer non-chemical intervention, after having had a swab test and the results, seek the help of a professional medical herbalist. In the meantime be scrupulous about personal hygiene, wipe from front to back, avoid vaginal deodorants and perfumed lavatory paper, and wash the area simply with warm water with a little apple cider vinegar added to it. Wear cotton underwear and avoid anything tight, particularly support hose with a tight gusset. Ensure your diet is at its best.

VARICOSITY AND HAEMORRHOIDS

These are both the result of a body under stress as the result of a lack of nutrients. This causes weakness in the circulatory system so your first port of call is to improve your diet. You will find that the calcium tea will make a big difference straight away (see pages 51, 102). Foods high in vitamin C and bioflavonoids, such as rosehips and all the citrus fruits (you must include the white pith to get the advantage of bioflavonoids), and also foods high in rutin, especially buckwheat, will all help to strengthen fragile capillaries. A particularly wonderful buckwheat porridge can be made from sprouted buckwheat liquidised with stewed hunza apricots and a piece of fresh peeled ginger root. Obviously putting your feet up while resting and elevating the foot of the bed while sleeping will help as this encourages the blood to flow easily to the heart.

Make a double-strength decoction of white oak bark and soak support stockings in it and go to bed in these. If carried out faithfully for a week or so this really does help.

Haemorrhoids can be treated by applying ice cold witch-hazel on gauze over a swelling, by using pilewort ointment around and in the anus applied with a clean finger after every bowel movement and, best of all, by inserting a piece of raw potato cut to the size of the little finger into the rectum. This brings relief very quickly. Hot and cold sitz baths using cypress oil in the hot water, 20 drops to four inches (10 cm) of hot water is also very helpful. Sometimes it helps to roll up two small hand towels in the hot sitz bath and place one buttock on either hand towel, thus spreading them and allowing the cypress oil dissolved in the hot water to really reach the area.

A cloth dipped in a strong decoction of white oak bark and applied externally often can be very helpful for varicose veins which sometimes appear on the labia. If you are suffering from this problem do go and see an osteopath or a chiropractor who can check the tilt of your pelvic girdle which may be causing it.

• MORE SERIOUS DISEASES THAT MAY COMPLICATE PREGNANCY •

CHLAMYDIA

This is now one of the most prevalent sexually-transmitted diseases in the Western world. If you are pregnant a concern is that babies born to infected women may develop pneumonia. The problem with chlamydia is that in women there are usually no symptoms at all. You may detect some or none of these signs: a vaginal discharge ranging from a thin and white liquid to copious green and yellow, some vulval and vaginal soreness, sexual intercourse might be painful, and, very occasionally, urination may be painful or frequent. Your partner may get a sore on the urethra one or two weeks after contact, making it painful to urinate, as well as discharge from the penis and sometimes inflammation of the joints. If you have any worries that you might be infected with chlamydia it is preferable to get a genital swab taken before you become pregnant. If it is positive your doctor will be able to advise the best course of action. My approach would be to place a woman on frequent doses of antibiotic herbs especially echinacea, golden seal and garlic.

> *Please note you should not attempt to treat chlamydia without seeking professional help.*

CYTOMEGALO VIRUS (CMV)

CMV is a common infection among pregnant women and is passed by kissing or sexual intercourse. The virus can be found in urine, saliva, breast milk, semen and cervical mucus but nearly all pregnant women in the Western world have antibodies to CMV. Symptoms are normally extremely mild and the risk of severe congenital disease to the baby is high only in about 5 per cent of women when primary CMV infection is present. So it is very unlikely to cause problems. If it is of concern to you, again it is possible for your doctor to check for this infection.

GENITAL HERPES

The risk of transmission of genital herpes to your baby is highest if you have your first attack near the time of delivery. The risk is much less if you suffer recurrent herpes of the genitals. Babies who contract the herpes virus during birth may suffer central nervous system or eye damage or, very rarely, die. A woman who has active lesions in her vagina at the time of labour should opt for a caesarean. However, if the lesions are on the thighs, bottom or anal area, safe vaginal delivery will be possible with a skilled midwife. Women with a history of herpes should have cultures of the vagina taken every week from the thirty-fifth week of pregnancy onwards and a vaginal examination using a sterile speculum should be done at the onset of labour or if the membranes rupture early, to rule out the presence of lesions. I have been able to support women who have been predisposed to genital herpes before they conceive throughout their pregnancy with high doses of echinacea, the decocted root made as a tea, four cups daily, and should they have an outbreak powdered golden seal applied locally as a mini poultice is extremely effective. Genital herpes will flair up when resistance is low as the result of illness, fatigue, sunburn, severe physical friction or any other type of stress and so a tremendous amount of emotional support is needed throughout pregnancy

GONORRHOEA

Some doctors feel that pregnant women should be tested for syphilis and gonorrhoea the first pre-natal visit, and that those at high risk for sexually transmitted diseases should have another culture test for gonorrhoea as well as a test for chlamydia and syphilis later in the third trimester. Untreated gonorrhoea in a pregnant woman may result in an infection of the baby's eyes.

INFECTIOUS HEPATITIS

Viral hepatitis B is transmitted through the blood, vaginal secretions, semen, saliva and blood by-products and mothers infected with it can transfer the virus to their babies during birthing. Infectious hepatitis may trigger premature labour. It is possible to be tested for this – infected women generally show signs of lack of appetite, nausea, vomiting, fatigue, jaundice, abdominal distension and fullness.

TOXOPLASMOSIS

This is an infection caused by a parasite as the result of eating infected undercooked meat or by contact with cat droppings. It causes severe congenital malformations and may result in premature labour or the death of the foetus.

• OTHER WORRIES •

When I interviewed Dianne Bjarnson I asked her about some of the worries that women might have about serious complications during pregnancy. One of the prime concerns is vaginal bleeding which is not due to an an obvious miscarriage. Her feeling was that abruptio placenta (separation from the placenta) is almost impossible unless a woman falls down very, very badly. Her experience is that if a woman is nutritionally sound her placenta is normally firmly attached to the uterine wall and it is extremely unlikely to become detached during the last three months of pregnancy. Dianne feels that women who keep getting vaginal infections do so because the circulation in their vaginal areas diminishes as the result of self-induced tension. She prefers to do vaginal massage on her pregnant patients predisposed to a lot of vaginal discharge so increasing the circulation in the area. One of the added bonuses of this she noticed was a softening of even a really tough cervix making birthing easier.

Dianne felt that the problem of a small pelvis is highly over rated. Although some doctors claim they can predict whether a woman's pelvis will be too small to have a vaginal delivery they can't do so with certainty unless the pelvis is obviously deformed due to injury or rare and severe childhood nutritional disease. Years ago, during the industrial revolution when people's lives were disrupted by being forced to move to cities, live in poverty and suffer as a result from severe nutritional deficiency pelvic disproportion (cephalo-pelvic dispro-portion) may well have been a problem, but now it is acknowledged that even if a woman has a small pelvis her baby's head may be smaller than average or her pelvic bones may open wider than expected or the baby's head will mold and pass through the opening. Research done in a 1960s study proved this and as long as a woman's labour, however slow, does not stop, any progress indicates that the head of the baby is able to pass through the pelvis. Dianne herself has assisted many first-time mothers with so called small pelvis' to have successful vaginal births. She also feels that a dry labour is a very over-rated threat and that the amniotic fluid at the end of pregnancy often decreases. She observes that the stress of labour is harder on the placenta so that the baby does not get as much oxygen as possible but there is usually no problem if the baby and the mother are nutritionally sound or even fairly nutritionally sound because the baby is designed to handle stress during labour, as is the mother. She is happy to handle premature labour up to three weeks before birth but won't stretch it beyond that. She will assist women to have a vaginal birth after a caesarean and points out that uterine rupture occurs only once in every 1,500 births and that normally she can detect who might be predisposed to this by looking at their skin and the condition of their hair and nails. If hair and nails are poor and constantly breaking and the skin is very thin she prefers to send them to hospital but otherwise throughout pregnancy she encourages a woman to eat a nutritious diet and to massage olive oil, vitamin E oil and castor oil into the scar several times daily throughout pregnancy. She seldom runs into a problem with a prolapsed cord because she doesn't usually handle premature babies. Her feeling is that if the baby has reached full term and the head is well down a prolapsed cord is unlikely. She points out that one third to a quarter of all babies have cords around their neck and they have had for centuries and providing they are full term this is generally not a problem.

Another great fear of pregnant women is haemorrhage after birth which Dianne believes is greatly reduced by responsible nutrition throughout pregnancy. She also observes that relaxant drugs are not used during labour at a home birth and considers that if a woman is given such a drug it relaxes the uterus so much it stays after the baby is born and does not clamp down. This makes the mother more predisposed to haemorrhage. In cases of haemorrhage she uses shepherd's purse tincture with a great deal of success (see pages 20, 112).

In response to all the drugs used during a hospital birth she says, 'It is very common when I talk to nurses who have delivered babies in hospitals for them to think it is normal for a baby to come out with difficulties, eye problems, respiratory problems, etc., and I just point out it is all the drugs that have gone into the baby before it was born. Babies whose mothers are not drugged are healthier and livelier and do not have to be resuscitated as much at home. Women who work in the new-born nurseries can tell the difference between a baby whose mother has had an epidural and one who hasn't.'

• RISK FACTORS •

Many pregnant women are afraid of home births. They think a situation will suddenly arise during their labour or birth which might result in death or injury to the baby or themselves unless high technology is instantly available. In reality only extremely rare situations which could happen suddenly are serious enough to potentially cause death or injury either to you or your baby. These are a prolapsed cord, abruptio placenta, uterine rupture and the baby's shoulder getting stuck. Even in hospitals (where such complications might well be more likely to happen due to unnecessary intervention) the incidence of any of these occurring are *very low indeed*. In almost every instance in which a woman without a previous history of caesareans has had a uterine rupture it has occurred in conjunction with a difficult delivery due to obstetrical interference such as artificial induction of birth, internal rotation of the foetus, or pulling out the baby in a breech position. Realistically the chance of a woman who has not had a previous caesarean having a uterine rupture at home is *so slight and so far outside the experience of even the most experienced midwife that it is beyond consideration.*

Certainly of the hundreds and hundreds of babies that Dianne has delivered over the years she has not encountered it once. In the very rare instance of a prolapsed cord, a baby's shoulder getting stuck or abruptio placenta there are emergency measures which can be taken at home by a skilled midwife or on the way to a hospital until medical care is available.

CHAPTER 6:

GIVING BIRTH AND THE IMMEDIATE POST-NATAL PERIOD

———

• HERBAL TREASURE CHEST FOR BIRTH •

The last few weeks before your due date is an excellent time to gather together all the herbs your baby and you will need during the birthing process and immediately afterwards.

Research which has been going on since the 1980s now indisputably proves that babies in the womb begin to use their senses eight weeks after conception, beginning with the sense of touch and going on to the sense of taste and smell. By twenty-four weeks in utero they are capable of learning, by twenty-six weeks of detecting light, and by thirty-six weeks they can recognise familiar sounds. So it is a good idea to prepare the birthing room so that when your baby emerges the environment is both reassuring and familiar. For a few weeks before the birth tune into your favourite music on a regular basis, stroking your tummy and reassuring the baby that everything is alright is helpful too. If you play the same music while in labour this will reduce the contrast between the womb and the outside world for the baby. Burn the same essential oils you will be using in the delivery room in an oil diffuser and in this way all the senses will become inextricably linked in your baby's mind: music, reassurance, relaxation and aroma. Essential oils in the delivery room don't simply fragrance it, but cleanse the air and provide a familiar welcoming aroma for the baby. You can dab them on a cotton wool ball and place them under your pillow or on a radiator, or you can dilute them and burn them in an oil diffuser. Lavender, neroli, maroc rose or geranium will make excellent oils for this purpose. **Lavender** is calming, smells sharp and clean, and when inhaled is excellent for headaches, shock or fainting. **Neroli** relaxes you by increasing the oxygen supply to the blood and so will stop you hyperventilating. In low doses it has a slightly sedative effect; at higher doses it acts as a stimulant. One to two drops diluted in 5 ml of carrier oil in an oil diffuser is enough to be effective. The fragrance of **rose oil** can be overwhelmingly sweet to some, so do check that you like it before you buy. It has a slightly analgesic effect and is a good cardiac tonic. **Geranium oil** is very up-lifting and just inhaling its fragrance will help to promote good circulation and so make breathing easier.

Some women have said to me that having small tubs of these herbs growing in the delivery room is very helpful as they can pick them and crush them in their hands while in labour.

- For internal use blue cohosh tincture is my favourite birthing herb. Twenty drops two or three times a day if you are overdue will help to soften and ripen the cervix and usually works within a week. As an oxytoxic it is extremely good for haemorrhage as it actually clamps down the womb.
- **Cayenne tincture** is an absolute must. Get the strongest best quality you can find. Again it is excellent for bleeding but unlike blue cohosh does not actually contract the womb it merely controls bleeding; so for haemorrhage the best mixture of all is half and half blue cohosh and cayenne tincture. Cayenne tincture given neat on the tongue is excellent for shock. If a woman is exhausted and drifting it will bring her attention back to the present very rapidly. I advise mothers to make up the following excellent labour drink. Shock tea recipe (more p 119).
- **Red raspberry leaf tea** made as a double-strength infusion will help to expel the placenta. Some women say it cuts down the pain of contractions if sipped hot throughout labour and certainly it is rich in vitamin C and so helpful to stop stretch marks and relax tense breasts. As a single-strength infusion it is also wonderful for washing out a baby's eyes straight after birth. It should be done using a padded gauze not fibrous cotton wool.
- **Rescue remedy** The famous Dr Bach's Flower Remedy is useful for anyone who needs a bit of a boost including your partner, the midwife, or any doctors in attendance, as well as family members. Use 4 drops on the tongue as needed.
- **St John's Wort oil** I have used this many times with great success massaged into the lumbar sickle area for after-birth pains, coupled with doses of equal parts of lobelia and cayenne tincture given internally, 5 drops as needed.
- **Lobelia tincture** This is excellent for helping with after-birth pains (see above). Again mixed half and half with cayenne tincture, 20 drops in a little grape juice given during the first stage of labour as needed helps to make the labour milder but the other stages of labour much more efficient. Do not give this beyond the first stage. Occasionally Dianne tells me that she gives a lobelia tincture enema using 1 oz (30 g) of lobelia tincture to 2 pints (1¾ litres) of warm pure water. She uses an enema for women who have been in labour for a day who are absolutely pooped when they don't have the energy and they just need a little rest. This enables them to sleep between contractions for about half an hour and will really restore their energy again so this is a really useful aid. She will also give it to a

first time mother where the baby's head is too high. Her feeling is they need to clear out some blockage in the bowel in order for the head to move down and she has observed that diarrhoea is quite normal just before a woman goes into labour, indeed it is a sign of labour. If women don't experience diarrhoea and the baby's head is too high, she will use the lobelia enema to pull the faeces out of the body and so make the head come down further, putting pressure on the cervix and helping the cervix to work better.

● **Dr Christopher's prenatal formula** Mix equal parts of finally powdered squawvine, blessed thistle, black cohosh, penny royal, false unicorn, raspberry leaves and lobelia together. Take three size 00 capsules morning and evening. This is an excellent formulation for giving elasticity to the pelvic and vaginal areas and so strengthening the reproductive organs for easier delivery but it should only be taken consistently in the last 6 weeks before the baby is expected. I have used this for many years with a great deal of success. Occasionally if the labour is very slow and the woman needs some assistance the contents of three capsules opened up and stirred into a little warm water will accelerate matters.

● **Siberian Ginseng tincture** This is useful for helping sustain energy and to slow down early contractions.

● **Castor oil** Some women mix this in orange juice and take it to start contractions and interestingly the contractions will stop if it is not time to give birth.

NB If you have problems during pregnancy castor oil can cause premature births so it is not to be taken in this instance. A safer approach would be to rub it on to your tummy or (see above) to take an increased dose of pre-natal formulation by doubling it morning and evening if you think you are overdue.

● **Calcium tea** (see page 51, 102) If you are hypoglycaemic or suffering from gestational diabetes as birthing will often exacerbate low blood sugar the day after the birth try and drink several pints of this each day for several days after the birth if needed.

● **Shepherd's purse tincture** This is another wonderful styptic, that is it will stop internal and external bleeding during childbirth. See also the section on cayenne tincture.

● **Comfrey leaf** Used as a poultice it will help to heal and mend episiotomies. Do not use the root which can be very drawing and make the whole area break down into uncomfortable bumps. Comfrey leaf poultices applied hot to cracked nipples will both sooth and heal.

● **Sitz bath herbs** Gather the following herbs together in equal quantities and put them in a muslin draw-string bag for use either as a sitz bath after labour for the mother or as the baby's bath herbs to rub the body down after the birth.

Equal parts: Myrrh gum powder, sea-salt, comfrey leaf, uva ursi, shepherd's purse, lavender and rose petals. Make a decoction, allow to cool to body temperature and use as needed.

- **Golden seal powder and Myrrh powder** Both are antiseptic and healing sprinkled onto the stump of the baby's cut umbilical chord.
- **Elderflower, peppermint and composition essence** (see Resources Directory). In hot water, sipped as needed, will cut down the transition time in labour.
- **Pregnancy tea** I hope that you have been faithfully drinking your pregnancy tea (see page 100) throughout your pregnancy because during labour is when it really comes into its own and pays off. It will help you to have a much easier labour.

Dianne Bjarnson's cervix softening formula

Dianne uses this with great success, particularly on first-time mothers where labour tends to be longer. Not only does it soften the cervix and make it riper but it has the added advantage of helping women with a predisposition towards high blood pressure not to convulse during labour while actually bringing the blood pressure down.

8 parts of rice bran syrup (Bernard Jensen makes an excellent one in America but it is not available in Europe) or blackstrap molasses
2 parts cayenne tincture

2 parts lobelia tincture
2 parts blue cohosh tincture
2 parts ladies slipper tincture or 2 parts hops tincture.

NB Ladies slipper is specifically indicated to relax the os of the cervix but unfortunately it is now an endangered species so hops is an acceptable substitute.

This formulation should be taken during the last four weeks of pregnancy half a teaspoon in the morning and at lunchtime, one teaspoon before bed. The only women who should not take it are those with a family history of very short labours.

• THE BIRTH •

Remember the atmosphere you create, the environment and the attenders at your birthing are entirely your choice. It is also your privilege to change your mind about what you have chosen even at the very last minute. Don't be afraid to do this. If you already have children, depending on the atmosphere within your family and its previous traditions, you may like them to be there to watch the actual birthing of the new addition to the family or to be invited in shortly afterwards once you are covered up. Most of my pregnant patients do not like children in the room during the process of labour as they need all their concentration for the contractions. Bear in mind some children don't like the sight of blood although in my experience most are not squeamish if confronted with a little. Interestingly, when children are present shortly after the birth, a real bonding tends to take place and there is less sibling rivalry and jealousy. This may well make for good babysitters in the future!

The whole purpose of a vaginal birth is so that the baby gets massaged as she comes down the vaginal canal helping lymph, blood, heart, brain and diaphragm as well as clearing the lungs and regulating and nourishing the cells. Babies who are born vaginally have to be resuscitated far less than ones born by a caesarean section. If there has been any meconium in the amniotic fluid (the result of a bowel movement from the baby) a midwife will normally suction the mouth of a baby and then the nose.

The amniotic fluid, which in 85 per cent of births comes out when the cervix is fully dilated and the mother begins to push, is normally clear and straw coloured. If it is stained dark yellow or green it could be because the baby has had a bowel movement inside the uterus. This is considered a risk factor as 5 per cent of babies who are born with meconium-stained amniotic fluid die as opposed to only 1 per cent who don't have it. Babies in a breech position always pass meconium simply because their buttocks are pressed against the dilating cervix which forces the meconium out and this is certainly not a cause for concern, but in other instances the commonly accepted explanation is that babies have a bowel movement if they are head down when they are under stress due to oxygen deprivation.

In itself meconium does not hurt the baby unless it breaths in some of the thick sticky material, in which case there is a danger of blocked airways and subsequent lung infection. Hence the reason for suctioning a baby's mouth and then nose in this situation. Dianne will leave the baby in the vaginal canal for a further contraction with its head out because this will squeeze the chest and bring everything out naturally from the baby's mouth and nose. She observes that if a woman is two weeks overdue there may be some meconium in the water and that if her vaginal discharge is bright yellow this would indicate the possibility of meconium staining so she, as a midwife, is prepared for it.

Only once in twenty years of home deliveries has she had to transport a baby to hospital because of meconium aspiration. It didn't contract pneumonia because, even though the breathing was high, within a day the baby had had an enormous bowel movement and after that everything seemed to calm down very quickly. Once again in this instance the mother took very good care of herself during pregnancy, particularly nutritionally.

Juliet de Bairacli-Levy, a revered and now a very elderly herbalist observes in her book, *Nature's Children* that animals fast before they give birth and that she herself did so before the birth of her two babies. As a result she noticed an immediate speedy and powerful release of energy available for the birthing process itself. She also advises fasting for a few days after the birth taking in only liquids and cold-water bathing immediately after birth. I haven't ever been able to persuade any of my pregnant patients to do this but I have observed that the heavy food served in hospital immediately after birth can result in a lot of pain, discomfort and vomiting. My advice is if you are not having a baby at home take in your own food and juices. Women when they do go into labour normally don't want to eat and this is quite a natural process encouraging their digestive system to shut down because all the energy is needed in the uterus.

Comfrey sitz baths can be very useful just before labour encouraging circulation into the perineal area, toning it and making it much more stretchy and elastic. As a little girl in Africa I observed women squatting over steaming hot rocks in order to soften up the perineum before birth. Normally a baby will come in a time that is right for her and should not be hurried. If there is real reason to hurry her along you could resort to the measure suggested on pages 115–116.

• PAIN CONTROL DURING LABOUR •

The most effective methods of pain control I have observed, apart from learned breathing, hypnotherapy, visualisation and acupressure is birthing under water. For this the temperature of the water should be 37 to 39°C (99 to 101°F), just a little bit higher than body temperature and the water should be heated up beforehand, not by an electric heater in the water. It is important that the temperature is kept high enough so it is not a shock to the baby's system. The air around the bath and in the room in general should be kept very warm, so much so that it may feel uncomfortable and overheated to the attenders, but as the mother's shoulders will usually be projecting above the water, it is essential that all of her is kept warm.

• HERBS FOR LABOUR •

Make sure that you have these already in the house or take them into the hospital with you. Tinctures are preferable to teas in labour as they work much more quickly, particularly if added to a hot liquid.

Shock Tea for Labour

Mix a cup of warm water with two tablespoons of organic apple cider vinegar, an eighth of a cup of honey or organic maple syrup and a full teaspoon of cayenne powder.

This distinctive but quite tasty brew will stop the onset of any shock as well as warming the body by increasing the circulation, it will also raise blood sugar to provide energy and prevent any danger of haemorrhage. It can be drunk ad-lib throughout the birth to give energy. If the taste of cayenne gets too strong simply sip it through a child's bendy party straw.

I always ensure there is also a bottle of Bach Flower Rescue Remedy on hand and there are specific reflexology points that can be pressed to help with pain. Use the right foot during labour and the left to expel the placenta.

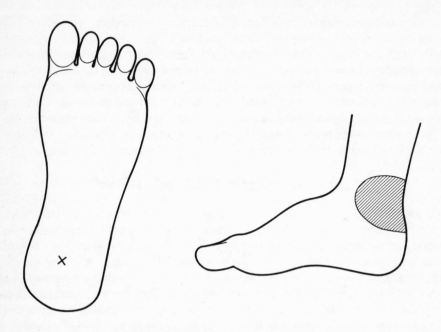

Reflexology points to facilitate labour

It can also be helpful to press the tines of combs on the fingertips, on the pads just below the fingers or across the heals of the hand. Alternatively you can get someone to work the comb over your skin for you. It is not uncommon for a labouring mother to get through four pints of the shock tea during labour and it is normally experienced as very welcoming, although, in other circumstances, it can taste rather strong.

A good invigorating overall foot massage on the soles and the top of the feet or a whole body massage can help resume sluggish contractions. The point located in the middle of the heel is a specific acupressure point used to facilitate contractions. Lady's Slipper tincture is indicated for loosening up a rigid cervix but, as it is an endangered species, it is difficult to get hold of. Administer ten drops every three minutes in hot water until it has completed its task.

• ENERGY HERBS DURING LABOUR •

Besides the shock tea, grape and apple juice are excellent for giving strength and ginger tea is specific for the female organs being both tasty and stimulating.

However, because it brings blood into the uterine area it should not be taken too close to the time of actual birth because it may increase the possibility of haemorrhage. Siberian Ginseng can give sustenance and strength during labour. Take 40 drops hourly.

Some of the pain experienced during labour is exacerbated by fear and tension. Coaching by an attentive birth attendant can help. I have known some women who believe that by relaxing their mouth they can affect the dilation of the cervix. Some women find relief from pressure applied on the sacrum or femoral bones. Dianne has observed an enema of lobelia tea (1 oz/30 g) decocted in one pint (600 ml) of water and strained can cut the pain by half. In the early part of labour, when the contractions ache like menstrual cramps, motherwort tincture can reduce some of the pressure. Take five drops in warm water as needed. Later on in labour scullcap or St John's Wort, or both mixed together, taken ad-lib work well for decreasing the pain.

When you are pushing don't be afraid to grunt or moan or call out because the feeling of pushing a baby can be the most intense experience you have had. Vocalising it is fine. Some women cannot feel the baby descending the birth canal clearly but when the vaginal opening bulges and the top of the head appears you will be told to stop pushing while the perineum is supported and pant lightly, pushing gently as the head emerges. When it does your birth attendant will immediately check for the cord around the neck and if it is there they will be able to pull it either around a shoulder or off the top of the head. Your birth attendant will let you know when it is time to expel the rest of the baby which usually happens in a soft swift swooshing movement. After the baby has fully emerged your midwife or doctor will usually examine it carefully to make sure the baby is generally fine and ensure the complexion changes from a bluish colour to a nice healthy pink. When they are convinced the baby is all right they will place it on your tummy for you to love and hold until the cord has stopped pulsating completely. At this point be sure to cover the baby with a receiving blanket. Remember the baby is going from 37°C (98.6° F) inside you to a 21°C (70° F) room temperature and is wet and slippery besides so will be very grateful for your body warmth.

The cord should stop pulsing completely before it is clamped and cut. Once the baby is washed and dressed put her diaper on in such a way that nothing touches her cord stump. Every time you change her you will need to replace the gauze pad by cutting a slit in the middle of it and slipping it over the cord stump and sprinkling a little golden seal or myrrh powder over the stump.

● PERINEAL CARE ●

While active labour often follows no preset pattern, it is generally thought that if the contractions increase in duration and decrease in time in-between you are in true labour, but many women I know have had irregular contractions and are still progressing rapidly. Some labours will begin with a bloody show, i.e. blood-tinged mucus. If the water breaks, labour usually begins, but sometimes if this happens labour doesn't start for some time after.

You can go for about four days after the premature rupture of the membranes without an increased risk of infection but if you decide you are happy watching and waiting make certain that you keep yourself fastidiously clean. You can take a teaspoon of half garlic and half echinacea tincture internally to reduce the risk of infection every two hours. Be sure to wipe yourself from front to back. If your water hasn't broken you can take a good hot bath if you suspect you are in labour. True labour will continue while a false labour will subside. Before you climb into the bath, it should be thoroughly scrubbed and disinfected. After giving birth every time you use the bathroom flush the perineal area with a combination of a pint of warm water and a teaspoon of goldenseal tincture. Again, always wipe from front to back and if you are torn or puffy and feel sore vaginally take plenty of comfrey leaf tea internally and wash externally over the area often. Gently dribble into the mouth of the vagina fresh aloe vera juice with a douche kit but do not insert the douche nozzle more than an inch into the vagina and be sure to use a fresh sanitary pad every time you use the bathroom. You will usually find nursing the baby will bring gushes of blood out and completely soak sanitary towels. Help in the first two or three weeks from a friend or relative while you nurse the baby is as vital as help during labour. In our modern busy world mothers are often left to get on with things as best they can far too soon after the birth.

• EPISIOTOMIES •

In Dianne's extensive experience if the partner or midwife gently massages the perineum with olive oil, applies warm compresses and guides the birthing movement gently, most women can stretch adequately to accommodate the head and bodies of their babies and even if some small tearing does occur it is often much less extreme and will mend more easily than the cut from an episiotomy. The massage should begin some weeks before the baby is due. St John's Wort, comfrey or arnica oil applied over the stitches of an episiotomy in gentle gauze poultice form will accelerate its healing as will cold sitz baths taken daily.

• THE PLACENTA •

Nursing the baby will stimulate contractions and help the expulsion of the placenta. Once it arrives, and this can take as long as an hour after the birth so don't panic if it does take time, your birth attendant will check thoroughly because if any placenta is retained you can develop a high fever which may endanger your life. If the placenta takes a while to expel drink a cup or two of red raspberry tea sweetened with plenty of honey and nurse the baby or stimulate the nipples as this powerfully contracts the uterus. I have also used Dong Quai to help expel the placenta in a decoction form sweetened with honey at the same dose.

If you feel like getting up to take a shower by all means do so but some women feel too weak to walk around right after a birth in which case don't bathe. Someone will give you a bed bath hopefully which feels wonderful if you have sweated hard during labour.

● AFTER-BIRTH PAINS ●

With some women liberal doses of St John's Wort tincture massaged externally on the inside of the thighs and lower spine can be helpful but I have found the deep heat oil (see page 115) massaged externally together with liberal doses of equal parts of cayenne and lobelia tincture in fruit juice very helpful. While you pass lochia, the bloody discharge that cleanses the body after birth, rest as much as you can, preferably in bed. Remember comfrey tea is a cell proliferant and will help to rebuild your body. Your diet at this point should include plenty of raw food and freshly made juices.

● POST-NATAL DEPRESSION ●

There are two good commercial products that I have used with success for post natal depression. The first is hyperisan and the second valerinnum zincum, both available from Bioforce. Instructions come on the package as far as the dosage is concerned. Sore stitches can be helped by fomentations of aloe vera juice or poultices of comfrey leaf provided the wound is not leaking any moisture. Hot and cold sitz baths also help with lavender oil added to the hot water, 10 drops to 4 inches (10 cm) of hot water in a basin.

● NURSING ●

A baby's blood glucose begins to drop at birth but will immediately rectify itself if nursed straight after birth. The longer nursing is delayed the more severe the drop becomes and a baby who is withheld from feeding for eight hours or more suffers severe hypoglycaemia which is extremely difficult to recover from. Breast-fed babies take in less volume of milk but they absorb and utilise the milk much better so they don't need ounce for ounce the same amount that bottle-fed babies do. Moreover mother's milk is more concentrated at birth and becomes much more watery as the baby grows which provides the perfect ratio of nutrients to liquid that a growing baby needs.

THE IMPORTANCE OF BREAST-FEEDING

It prevents poorly developed dental arches, pallets and other facial collapses in adulthood because breast-feeding babies encourages good facial and dental development. It prevents anaemia in both mother and baby because iron is infinitesimal in cows' milk. Breast-fed babies are less likely to suffer from eczema, allergies, infections, constipation and obesity. It has been shown that women who breast-feed get less breast cancer than those who don't. Nursing stimulates the release of hormones from the pituitary gland that help the uterus to return to its non-pregnant size and burn off excessive fatty tissue and, of course, it hardly needs to be said that the emotional bonding that develops between a mother and a child through breast-feeding creates a tremendous amount of love and trust.

The good news is that breast milk can convey natural medicine to a baby and I have treated very young babies in this way many, many times with a great deal of success. The bad news is that women eating hormones hidden in meat, pesticides, additives and preservatives pass these on to a baby who in her first year is still very vulnerable and whose brain, endocrine glands and other vital tissues are developing.

Happily there are specific ways a pregnant woman can minimise the risk to her baby. The less dairy products, eggs and fish you consume the less toxic chemicals will be found in your breast-feeding milk. In fact in 1976 the EPA analysed the breast milk of vegetarian women and discovered the levels of pesticides in their breast milk to be far less than average. A follow up study in the *New England Journal of Medicine* published 26 March 1981 confirmed that, 'The highest levels of contamination in the breast milk of vegetarians was lower than the lowest level of contamination in non-vegetarian women. The mean vegetarian levels were only 1 or 2 per cent as high as the average levels in the United States.' This is a hugely telling and important statistic. As yet, to my knowledge, no studies have been done on the breast milk of vegan women, but there is every likelihood that their milk would be many times safer than even their vegetarian cousins.

It is as well to remember that all women who may consider sometime in the future breast-feeding a baby should realise that the diet that they eat on a daily basis will greatly affect the health of that baby. Any chemicals that they ingest, but particularly pesticides, will be stored in their body's fatty tissues until it is released into milk and the concentration level of pesticides in milk is extremely crucial. The Environmental Defence Fund has proved that the average American baby which is breast-fed receives one hundred times more PCBs, on a body-weight basis, than the average adult. Couple this with the fact that the baby's immature liver is completely incapable of detoxifying these chemicals and you have yet another sound reason as to why I espouse a vegan diet.

Babies are resilient but for optional health of your child you still need to be very careful about what you eat and drink.

POSITION OF THE BABY

Never nurse a baby while she is lying flat on her back from the breast or the bottle. The nasal cavity and the mouth both connect to the back of the throat which leads in turn to openings in the middle ear and if these get flooded with any kind of liquid it can result in recurring middle-ear infections, chronic nasal discharge and allergies. If you are using a bottle you must hold it in your hand and not prop it against your baby's face. The pressure from the bottle leaning against the baby's mouth can deform the growing jaw and teeth. Ensure that the hole in the nipple is large enough so that when the bottle is turned upside down milk drips easily from it because excessively hard sucking on the baby's part can lead to stomach distension.

NIPPLES

I have already discussed the proper care and preparation of nipples on pages 89–90 but to minimise stress upon them during nursing alternate your breasts. Make sure that the baby takes enough of the nipple and areola into her mouth while nursing. Insert a finger into the corners of the baby's mouth to break the baby's suction on your breast at the end of each nursing session. If you get a breast infection apply hot poultices of mullein and lobelia to the breast and do make sure that you are getting plenty of calcium in the form of calcium tea (see pages 51, 102). Also take plenty of liquids and hot baths and get lots of rest because many breast infections are the result of exhaustion. You shouldn't suffer from any engorgement if you nurse from the time of birth onwards. A hot ointment such as tiger balm or the deep heat oil massaged specifically into the area that hurts can be tremendously comforting.

If your breast milk isn't flowing adequately drink a tea made of four parts of fennel and two parts of blessed thistle. Decoct and drink four cups a day. If you need to decrease the flow of breast milk sage or parsley tea are very helpful.

Ideally you should aim to breast-feed for six months and your baby will let you know if she is in need of more than breast milk by beginning to chew your nipples. Interestingly Chloe Fisher, a leading midwife in Oxford, says that she has been able to correct 99 per cent of problems with sore nipples by correctly positioning the baby at the breast. Ensure that your nipple is centred in the baby's mouth with as much of the underside taken in as the upperside, and as mentioned previously, get as much of the aerola into the mouth as possible. Raspberry leaf tea helps to relax tense breasts and make them more flexible, as does massage with olive oil and comfrey ointment is very comforting for cracked nipples.

For toddlers who simply won't let go of the nipple because it gives them so much satisfaction and the mother is exhausted I have managed to discourage breast feeding by getting the mother to rub a mixture of penny royal and myrrh tincture into the nipples encouraging the mother to leave it on while the two year old latched on to the breast. The bitter taste soon put her off without making her feel too upset.

SOYA MILK

As far as soya milk is concerned soya infant formulations have been used for decades and there has not, to date, been a single report of adverse effects. There have been hundreds of studies on the effects of soya and apart from a few that illustrated an allergic reaction, almost all others have shown highly beneficial effects. Bear in mind that whilst soya-bean consumption may be relatively new in the Western world, Asian countries have eaten soya-bean foods for centuries. There have been no reports of any toxic effects there. Remember that cows' milk is loaded with oestrogen and that these are not mild ones derived from plants but potent ones from another mammal, the long-term effects of which we have yet to grapple with.

The concern about soya beans is that they contain isoflavones or phytoestrogens which act like oestrogens. Although these isoflavones are very weak (between 1,000 and 100,000 times weaker than oestrogen) the soya bean contains high concentrations and so people eating soya products tend to have higher concentrations in their blood. In adults isoflavones have the remarkable effect of not increasing oestrogen activity but instead of actually normalising oestrogen levels. Most women who eat the standard Western high-fat diets already have high levels of oestrogen in the bloodstream which is known to increase the risk of breast cancer. The isoflavones stop the oestrogen from exerting their effect at promoting cell division and so actually protect women from breast cancer. In 1994 there were more than 200 scientific papers dealing with the anti-cancer effects of eating soya food. Women on very low-fat diets sometimes have abnormally low levels of oestrogen which can result in risks to their reproductive functioning and bone strength. In this instance soya foods raised the oestrogen activity.

Don't be in too much of a hurry to give supplementary bottles. This is something some mothers do because they question their own ability to produce enough milk. Your body responds to the baby's demands. If you start to give bottles the baby takes less milk from you and so you will in turn produce less and have to give more bottles and so the vicious cycle goes on. If you really want to breast-feed simply persevere and feed your baby on demand trusting yourself and nature. Babies have very different requirements to adults and so ordinary cows' milk and soya milk that children and adults drink is not suitable for babies. Soya milk should not be given to babies under two years old because the fat level is too low and the protein content too high. Cows' milk is also too high in protein and is unsuitable for babies under one. If you want to bring your child up as a vegan there are several baby milk formulations made with soya beans which are specifically designed for babies and are safe. They have a higher fat content which meets the needs of growing babies and a protein level which conforms to the government health regulations for infants feeding.

WEANING

Getting your baby to switch from an all-milk diet, whatever its source, to one that includes solid food is a process that some mothers view with dread. But the weaning process is really a very simple one and most babies accomplish it smoothly. If you are contemplating bringing up your baby a vegetarian or vegan the weaning process should be along the following lines.

Between four to six months old

Give your baby a little fresh unsweetened fruit juice, diluted half and half with boiled filtered water which is first cooled. Suitable juices include orange (freshly squeezed, but frozen or unsweetened and non concentrated from a carton will do) or apple from a carton fortified with vitamin C but without any other additives. If you have a history in your family of intolerance to citrus fruits avoid oranges. Feed this fruit juice initially from a teaspoon in the middle of the morning or the afternoon and as soon as the baby gets used to taking it in this way try to give it from a normal cup and not from a mug with a feeder. This is the ideal way to introduce her to a cup and in the interim continue with breast or bottle feeding in the normal way.

Rest assured breast milk supplies all she needs including vitamin C for the first six months so if she is happy and thriving don't even contemplate introducing any solids until she is six months old. However if at four months she is not fully satisfied with your milk or with bottled milk, you might try giving a first taste of food. Don't start before four months old as the danger of introducing solids to an immature digestive system may result in an allergic reaction which you certainly don't want. The first spoonfuls of any food you feed are simply to get the baby used to the taste and feel of solid food and can't be regarded as nourishment. The baby still needs milk feeds for that and the emotional satisfaction of sucking. The first taste of solid food should be half a teaspoon of fruit or vegetable puree. Don't go for cereals as these can often cause allergies if given so early. While you may worry about possible allergic reactions when introducing your baby to a range of new foods these are actually fairly rare and when they do occur are often genetically passed down so you will have some idea that they may crop up if you know your family's history. Delaying solid food until your baby is six months old greatly reduces the risk of allergic reaction because the digestive system is much more mature and so able to cope. The most common foods to cause allergies are milk and any other dairy products, nuts, eggs, certain fruits and foods containing gluten which includes all grains except for rice and millet. The signs of an allergic reaction are rashes, swelling of the eyes, lips and face, sickness, diarrhoea, hay fever and asthma or eczema. In general babies will often outstrip their allergies by the time they are two years old although the allergy to dairy products can last for life as can one to nuts.

If you are planning to go back to work but want to continue to breast-feed, start giving the solids at lunch-time as this will eventually become the first meal at which the baby gives up breast-feeding and has only solids. In general it is better to offer solids before the milk feed so that you can gradually increase the quantity until your baby is satisfied and eventually dismisses the milk but there is no point in trying to give solids if the baby is hungry, wanting comfort and crying for a feed. Better to feed first and give solids second.

To do this use a shallow flat spoon and don't be offended if she spits out your offering. She is not being personal and remember there is no hurry. If there is a history of allergies including asthma, hay fever and eczema try one food for at least four days before introducing another, keeping a careful eye on your baby for any reaction. You can gradually aim to increase the quantity so that after a few weeks she is having up to two tablespoons at a time so allowing her tender digestive system to adapt slowly. Vegetables such as carrot, swede and parsnip puree can be prepared by boiling in a little unsalted filtered water until tender and then pureeing with a touch of water to make it soft. Apple puree can be made in the same way but use sweet apples not tart ones. The same applies to pears. If using bananas remove the seeds with the point of a knife and mash the flesh thoroughly with a fork adding a little cooled boiled water to achieve a softer consistency. Avocado is one of my favourite and very nutritious. Simply cut it in half, scoop out the flesh and mash it adding a few drops of boiled water if desired. When preparing tomatoes, sieve cooked ones to remove the seeds and scald and peel raw ones, cutting out the core and then mashing.

Pears, apples, peaches, apricots, nectarines, sweet cherries, plums, mangoes and kiwi fruit can all be eaten raw once the skin and pips are removed and they are mashed thoroughly. Broccoli, cauliflower, Brussels sprouts and cabbage of all colours can create intestinal gas and if this is a problem mix it with something blander such as carrot or parsnip. Only serve spinach once or twice a week because the acid content may affect the body's absorption of certain minerals. All dried fruit is fine but make sure it is unsulphured and not rolled in glucose and puree it until it is tender. Remember it can have a laxative effect. Once you get around to introducing cereals go for rice cereal first which is the least likely to cause an allergic reaction. If using corn, peas, green beans, avoid anything from a tin as these are very highly salted.

From six months onwards a little crushed wholemeal bread can be added to vegetable purees but remember that the bran in 100 per cent whole grain bread and flour can be too laxative for babies and an 85 per cent grain bread with added wheatgerm can be preferable. If adding nuts or seeds to fruit, powder them finely in a liquidiser first.

Solids from six to eight months

Now you are entering the stage where the demand for breast milk will decrease and you will probably find it takes two or three days for your body to catch up with the baby's decreased demand so your breasts may feel rather full. Rest assured this transitional period will only last for a few days. You can now begin to enrich simple fruit and vegetable purees with vegetable protein ingredients including beans such as soya, red kidney, cannellini, butterbeans and orange lentils. Use home-cooked beans not canned ones which are too high in salt and boil very thoroughly before rinsing, draining and pureeing. If feeding beans in tomato sauce, choose a variety without preservatives or colouring and mash or puree them mixing with a little crumbled whole grain bread and boiled water to moisten. Tofu works brilliantly mashed with mixed vegetables or fruit purees and Tahiti and other nut butters also work well with vegetable or fruit purees. Adding a quarter of a teaspoon to the Superfoods is an excellent idea if done once a day. If using nuts and seeds, mill them or powder them in a blender. A clean electric coffee grinder works well for this, or buy ground almonds. If grinding your own mix together a wide range of nuts so that you get a full range of nutrients. Start with half a teaspoon stirred into fruit or vegetable purees.

Provided your baby isn't allergic to wheat, add wheatgerm to soya yogurt and cereal mixes for extra nourishment.

By the time your baby has reached about nine months the bedtime feed may well be the only one left and don't be in a hurry to wean the baby from the bliss of this. Once the baby begins teething, she might find it comforting to chew on something hard such as a piece of apple, raw carrot, bread or rusks, but never leave her alone with this type of food because of the danger of choking. If anything does unhappily get stuck in her throat be instantly alert and able to hook it out quickly with your finger or turn her upside down and smack her gently in the small of the back until she coughs it out.

Feeding from eight to twelve months

As she enters her first year, it is reasonable to suppose she might want to join you and the family by eating what you are eating but in pureed form. Make certain that her portion is not too highly seasoned or salted but do be adventurous with new flavours because it will make it possible for you to eat out with friends or in a restaurant.

• SUGAR •

We all eat far too much of this and babies crave for sweet things so remember. Sugar as well as being in food like syrups is also present in large quantities in sugars and jams. Once absorbed into the bloodstream in a rush the body produces large amounts of insulin. This can lead to hypoglycaemia and worse. Use instead dried and fresh fruit, date puree, natural fruit juices with no added sugar and jams which are sweetened with grape juice.

Honey

A small amount of organic honey can be used from twelve months onwards but I prefer even smaller amounts of black strap molasses. Honey is a very concentrated food and contains no fibre so it has the same disadvantages as sugar, although good quality honey contains natural antibiotics.

Processed, canned and packaged foods

These all contain artificial additives and a minefield of other nasties and shouldn't really be eaten at any age. They are particularly bad for babies because of the increased possibility of allergic reactions. Certain additives have been linked with hyperactivity and aggression in young children, so try to avoid them wherever possible.

Whole nuts

Whether they be unsalted or salted they can easily get lodged in a baby's throat and cause choking. Unsalted nuts can be given from about 5 to 6 years old onwards.

Caffeine

Remember this is present not only in coffee but in tea, chocolate and all cocoa products as well as cola drinks. It is a stimulant and in quantity can be highly addictive.

Deep fried foods

Fat is difficult for a baby to digest and why burden her vulnerable body with free radicals at such an early age.

Eggs

In my opinion these are not good for anyone at any age but doctors have warned that eggs fed to children under 2 years of age carry the risk of food poisoning unless they are well cooked, that is hard boiled.

Dealing with Tantrums

It is best to stick to foods you know will be eaten and so avoid battles at will. All children have to go through the stage when they learn the power of the word no and unfortunately this can often be given back to you. Sometimes offering two equally nutritious items instead of one can stop the veto. Babies like feeding themselves although they often don't use the right tools and eat food in the right order. Don't spoil their fun. If they want to splash it all over themselves simply use a good feeding bib that is washable or wipe downable and cover the floor in newspapers. This will mop up most disasters.

It simply isn't worth making an issue over food or allowing a difficult situation to build. Remember it is your relationship with your growing toddler that is most important and this needs to be put before the horrors of broken nights, tantrums, food fads or puddles on the carpet.

PART THREE:
BABIES AND TODDLERS

———

CHAPTER 7:
HEALTH ISSUES FOR BABIES AND TODDLERS

——

Babies from birth to six months

Babies do actually breathe in the womb so it is perfectly understandable, on emergence, that a baby might have some fluid in her lungs. If she is not premature she is perfectly capable of getting this normal mucus out of her lungs alone and you can expect her breathing initially to sound moist and a bit mucusy. She will cough and sneeze through the first few weeks of life clearing out her lungs and doing any invasive unpleasant thing to her with the purpose of stimulating her is unnecessary. A baby that is breathing well and has a good heart beat does not need to be stimulated. Even if she doesn't breathe in the first few moments of life she can still get oxygen from the umbilical cord as long as it is not cut.

JAUNDICE

About two-thirds of all newborns get a little jaundice and it is something all midwives, paediatricians and health visitors keep an eye out for. Simple jaundice begins around the second or third day after birth and can last for a week or ten days. It is the result of bilirubin coming from the fragmenting of old or extra blood cells and this is usually excreted through the liver bile into the intestinal tract. The kidneys will also handle a little of it. A new baby has a lot of extra red blood cells to break down and a liver which is a little immature and overloaded so she will take a few days to catch up. A newborn with simple jaundice is normally orange, pink or tanned, eats well and is alert. The colouring comes from deposits of bilirubin in the skin. Drink lots of catnip, comfrey or dandelion tea yourself and give a teaspoon of the tea several times a day to your baby. Ensure that your baby passes the meconium and if it doesn't come along within a day or two put yourself on the ICF No 1 and continue to breast feed. If it hasn't appeared by the third day there may be something wrong with the baby's digestive system so consult a doctor. Take your baby out into the sunlight naked for a few minutes every day or, if the weather is cold, sunlight is effective even if it comes through a window to break down bilirubin.

If your baby is very lethargic, feverish, will not feed and looks pretty yellow all over there is a chance that the jaundice is more serious and the levels of bilirubin may get so high that brain damage is caused. In this case you do need to consult your doctor.

Breast-milk jaundice is extremely rare and is caused by a hormone in the mother's milk which inhibits the enzymes needed for the breakdown and excretion of bilirubin. This jaundice is not life-threatening and you should simply stop breast feeding for a day at the most while taking two ounces (60g) of fresh wheatgrass juice and giving a few drops diluted in plenty of water to the baby. Sunlight works just as well as bilirubin lights (sometimes used in hospitals to simulate sunlight). The dangers of artificial lights include irritability, sluggishness, diarrhoea, intestinal upset, dehydration, feeding difficulties, riboflavin deficiency, disturbance of the bilirubin-albumin relationship, poor visual orientation with the possibility of diminished responsiveness to parents and DNA modifying effects. It is also now beginning to be suspected that the use of bilirubin lights might be responsible for increased mortality, particularly in newborns because of lung problems and haemorrhage.

The only really dangerous kind of jaundice is the result of Rh or ABO blood incompatibility, a liver which is malfunctioning, damaged or diseased in some way, or a side effect of something wrong with the mother including infection and drug use. If your baby isn't eating well and is very hard to rouse and doesn't generally look well you must seek urgent medical advice.

COLIC

Colic is the result of trapped wind in the intestines, generally the result of undeveloped but a rapidly growing digestive system. This is why it will often start at three weeks and then finish about eight or ten weeks later. I have never worked out why night-time colic will begin at about seven and finish almost like clockwork at ten o'clock at night but I assume it is a build up of wind over the course of the day.

Very young babies can get colic for reasons the distraught parents cannot ascertain so ensure that the baby is firmly handled and not fiddled around with, and is carried around with you either in your arms or in a sling as close bodily contact is very soothing. Ensure when feeding that the line of the baby's head and body is at a 60° angle to the floor and that the baby is never allowed to lie flat while drinking. An excess of vitamin-B_6 on the mothers part (dosage of over 100 mgs per day) can suppress lactation and cause nerve injury. Exposing both mother and baby to regular light is important to ensure adequate supplies of vitamin D in the breast milk and a vegan mother should take special care to ensure that she is getting plenty of B_{12} rich foods so that the extra B_{12} she is not storing in her own liver and muscles is available in the breast milk for her baby. One of the simplest and most obvious reasons for a baby becoming colicky is the failure of the nursing mother to drink plenty of fluids by way of purified water and fruit and vegetable juices. While nursing you should be drinking an ounce of fluid for every pound of your body weight. I once had a frantic phone call from a graduate in Ireland asking for help with her grandchild who was colicky and horribly constipated. The simple solution was to remind the mother to drink. She had forgotten to while breast feeding and hence the baby's difficulties.

Suspect food allergies if the baby is constipated, has dark marks underneath the eyes, is windy, has red cheeks and is sweaty while sucking and wakes up suddenly. Remember that all the food you eat the baby is receiving too through your breast milk, and that the most common allergens are animal milk products, especially cows' milk, eggs, chicken, citrus fruit or juices, tomatoes, soya products, corn, rye, oats and wheat. You can eliminate these one by one from your own diet (it takes three days to get the food element out of your system entirely) and see if the baby improves.

Alternatively you can do it the other way around by eliminating them all from your diet for several weeks and then introducing them back one by one and keeping a close eye on the baby to see her reaction. Foods that make you very windy can also do the same for your baby and cause her discomfort. These include cabbage, broccoli, Brussels sprouts, radishes, turnips, cauliflower, onions and garlic, peanuts, chocolate, soaked prunes and prune juice as well as herbal laxatives.

I've seen cranial osteopathy and osteopathy do miraculous things for colicky babies if there is a problem with the skeletal structure and sometimes a faulty ileo-caecal valve can cause colic. A reflexologist or an applied kinesiologist can teach you how to put this right yourself.

I've had great success with catnip and fennel tincture. Put thirty drops in a cupful of boiling water and allow it to cool to lukewarm so evaporating the alcohol before administering it by the teaspoonful or dropperful as needed. You can't overdo the dosage on this so simply give as much as the baby will take and hopefully in ten minutes or so the cramping will stop as will the crying. Soothing baths using camomile or linden blossom in a bath bag helps, as does massaging the spine with lobelia tincture. If the baby is more than three months old try slippery elm gruel. Not only does it get rid of mucus but it absorbs all sorts of toxins and wind from the digestive tract.

• THRUSH •

If your baby has thrush which you can detect by white spots on the sides of the mouth, a white tongue or a yeast rash anywhere on the body, wash the infected area three or four times a day with Raspberry leaf or black walnut tea. Use cotton wool buds to get into the mouth. Give the baby the special baby acidophilus available from Biocare letting them know how old your baby is so that they can give you appropriate instructions (see Resources Directory) and make sure that you yourself don't have candida (see pages 96, 97).

● DRUGS AND YOUR BABY ●

Remember that it is possible any drugs you take during pregnancy, birthing, lactation and, also, new research would indicate, even during the months before conception can have an adverse affect on your baby. Alcohol, nicotine and any chemical drug you can name can all get through the placenta and affect the foetus within minutes. Even pain-killing and anesthetic drugs used during labour can cause foetal anoxia (severe oxygen deficiency) caused by the depressant effect of the drug on the respiratory system. Babies deprived of oxygen in this way are born limp, bluish, unable to breath spontaneously and may need oxygen and resuscitation. Up to 65 per cent of the babies of mothers medicated with anathesia in this way show symptoms of anoxia, and hypoxia (severe anoxia) can cause brain damage to the baby or even death.

Even a simple aspirin takes nineteen days to eliminate from your system and will go on affecting the baby for at least this long. So you are best advised not to take any drugs at all during lactation unless your life is threatened, there is no alternative and what you are being offered is literally life saving. If this is the case you are best advised to stop breast-feeding and move over to infant formula soya milk, nut milk and carrot juice. If for some reason your baby has been drugged common sense will dictate to you that she will need much more warmth, extra contact, reassurance and nurturing until the drugs leave her system.

However breast-feeding does accelerate the excretion of dangerous substances. Twice as much radio activity for example is excreted from breast-fed babies exposed to it than bottle fed babies similarly exposed.

● EYES ●

Your baby's eyes should be washed out using gauze dipped in strained lukewarm raspberry leaf tea, twice daily. This is particularly important if you live in a polluted area. Apart from bathing your baby daily in tepid water to which you can add infused lavender or rose petals, dirty areas such as the face and hands can be washed down with the following mixture which it's useful to have on standby. Ten drops of essential lavender or rosemary or thyme or sage oil in one pint of purified warmed water with a desert-spoon of apple cider vinegar added. Excess can be stored in a Kilner jar in an airing cupboard and taken out, shaken, and used as needed. It is not necessary to use soap on babies skin. You can tie soft oatmeal into muslin bags and soak these in water (when squeezed they will produce a milky liquid) and rub this over the skin to clean it if necessary.

Don't use talcum powder on babies. (Talcum powder used on the genital area of women has been proven to cause cancer of the ovaries). Use a little corn flour or arrow root instead.

After a month introduce your baby to air and sun baths beginning by an open window in the warmest hour of the day and simply exposing her to natural light for about five minutes. Gradually increase this to an hour within a month. Obviously if the weather is inclement it's not sensible to do this. Gradually if the weather dictates and if the baby's skin gets more resilient you can place her in a cot on a shady porch or beneath a leafy tree. Rub the skin with olive oil thinned down with a little cider vinegar, half a teaspoon of the vinegar to a tablespoon of oil. Keep a close eye on your baby to ensure she doesn't burn and place her feet not her head towards the sun.

In hot weather and during illness it is perfectly acceptable to give babies water and herbal teas.

All bed clothes and clothing should be light, loose and 100 per cent cotton and if wool is used it should be over cotton not against the skin. Synthetic fabrics should not be used through life at all. They suffocate the skin.

Babies put closely in touch with nature benefit very much from such contact so let them touch flowers and leaves. Hold them up to see sunsets and starry nights, birds and animals. Sounds during the first few months should be kept low and soothing, no sudden noises. The vibrations that you give out as a mother are probably the most important influence of all. You will experience time and time again that if you are uptight your baby will notice and start getting upset. She can't nurse well if she is crying because her stomach is too tense and her breathing will be out of rhythm. She will swallow air and start getting even more upset. You need to teach her to calm down before she begins sucking. If you simply stuff a nipple into her mouth just to quieten her, both of you will have fallen into a bad habit. Stop if you want to love each other three years from now and teach her that if she wants something the best way to get it is to be kind and sweet.

Once a baby reaches about 8 lb (36 kg) in weight she can pretty much maintain her own body temperature and doesn't, at this stage, need to be overdressed. I always feel very sorry for babies who are larger and are puce in the face from being wrapped in too many layers of clothing. If you touch her hands and feet and they feel slightly cool but her neck or abdomen is comfortably warm, you have got it about right. Babies will lose about 5 per cent of their body weight in the first few days and then they will stabilise and gain about an ounce per day averagely, larger ones gaining faster than smaller ones. As long as your baby is gaining (girls tend to be smaller than boys) just relax and flow with it. Worrying will only create the wrong vibrations between you and put the baby off her food.

The Toddler

It was Winston Churchill who said, 'It is easier to win two wars than raise two children.' He was speaking from first-hand experience, but it seems to me we have often made child-rearing a much more complicated process than it need be. Dr Liley observed, 'From the apparently eternal form of human pregnancy we can induce that the first child born to early man over a million years ago had precisely the same in utero experience as children born today. However, the ex utero environment has altered. Proto-hominid's child was born into an environment so similar to the one that he had just left that he did not need clothing, diapers, playpens, toilet training, spoon feeding, cribs or any of the other paraphernalia we associate with infant care today . . . There would be no bottom rashes or routines or formulas and very little crying . . . This shows that many of the problems we have with our babies have been created by ourselves.' If we look at some of the world's oldest societies we see they encourage a closeness between mother and child during the day by being carried, and at night by sleeping together. Weaning is very gradual and breast milk is taken for as long as possible. Massage of babies was encouraged both for its psychological benefit to mother and child (the eye and physical contact encourage a valuable intimacy) and for its ability to straighten the child's limbs and exercise it with the additional bonus of absorption of vitamins from the oils used, particularly vitamin D. Tribal societies accepted a child as an adult-to-be from an early age and spent much time deliberately introducing the child to the world around it so creating an honoured place for the child within society. Interestingly, older societies began toilet training at a very much earlier age – in Japan when the baby was only three months old. In the West this is not done usually until a child can walk or talk, which increases the frustrations of child-raising and the dependence on consumer products, particularly disposable nappies.

• WETTING AND TOILET TRAINING •

Traditional tribal people do not seem to need absorbent, protective substances to use for nappies for very long as most introduce a very successful toilet-training programme at an early age. For those who do use something leaves, bark clay cloth, made particularly soft by pounding or rags, were used to absorb the child's wetness. Sphagnum moss was particularly popular in North America. It can absorb up to twenty-two times its own weight in water compared to six times that of a cotton nappy and has the additional bonus of antibiotic substances in it, hence the reason why it was used during both the first and second world wars for wound dressing.

Most traditional tribal societies trained babies, some like the New Guineans, the Koreans, the Peruvians and some tribes in India as well as the Japanese from the age of about three months. What they all commonly seem to do is make a hissing sound for urination and imitate the sound of defecation while holding the child over an appropriate vessel or on a particular place on the floor, usually at a set time each day. The Eskimos cue the child by blowing gently on its head and Eskimo children are toilet trained before their first birthday. What all these successful toilet-training habits have in common is consistency of sound, regularity and encouragement. I suspect that our warnings in the West about early toilet-training creating psychological problems may well be a myth to protect the nappy industry.

Juliette de Bairacli-Levy opines, 'I think that the infant should be trained almost from birth to excrete into a receptacle, and not to lie on its back and soil itself. Only the child of man and the offspring of the pig and rodents soil themselves. It takes much time and patience to train an infant not to soil itself, but it is very worthwhile and saves time later on. The baby will usually secrete on waking from sleep and after meals, therefore he should be held over a chamber pot at these times. Urination is, of course, more difficult to control, being more frequent and irregular in timing, and infants cannot be trained to be dry. I used to pad my children's diapers with sheets of absorbent paper or with old soft cloths which I could burn and whenever possible they lay in the cradle without wearing napkins, bedded on that absorbent herb, sphagnum moss.' She notes that the Arabs used a sheepskin, woolly side uppermost, to place beneath babies in the cradle which could be washed easily and dried speedily and this is a wonderful addition to have in bed with you as the baby sleeps by your side (see Resources Directory). She also used powdered orris root or very finely powdered oatmeal to prevent skin chaffing, but I prefer cornflower or arrow-root.

• SOLID FOODS •

There can be no fixed rule for weaning. The time factor depends on each individual child and mother. Hopefully your child will be satisfied with your breast milk for at least the first six months and ideally this should be the earliest age that any food other than mother's breast milk should be introduced, but always remember that every baby is different.

Begin with one food only at a time and continue with this for at least a week. In this way it is easy to see if your baby can't handle that particular food or develops nappy rash. In which case you can eliminate it and try another one. Start with diluted juices. Freshly pressed carrot and apple juice are ideal, but don't mix fruit and vegetable juices at the same feeding because the enzymes in them are different. Within a few weeks you can begin to experiment with liquefied fruits and vegetables which can be processed in your blender. Ideally organic, ripe and in season. See also the advice on slippery elm which is the ideal weaning food on page 160. The most important consideration should be never to force-feed a baby or child. When children become ill they automatically stop eating, which is usually a healthy response, but do ensure they still get plenty of fluids until their body recovers and the appetite reappears spontaneously.

I have seen some right royal (and extremely painful) battles going on at the dinner table about food with children. The vital thing to remember is that every baby and child will do not what you *tell* them to do but copy what they *see* you doing. So the way to introduce a child to solid foods is to eat excellent whole natural foods yourself and, right from the word go, keep nothing in the house which you wouldn't want your child to eat. Also trust your child's instincts. I have never, in my many long years of clinical practice (and I have treated many thousands of babies and children), ever seen a child starve itself to death. Studies carried out with babies and small children show that provided they are offered only good high-quality foods, they are perfectly capable of choosing an excellent diet by themselves. It may look a bit erratic to adult eyes, peanut butter and bread one day and bananas the next, but a child's inner wisdom in choosing is superb. This does not apply if the diet on offer is one of processed chemicalised convenience foods. They create metabolic confusion in the body and a weakened immune system. I always thought the story of processed cereal v. the packet an apocrophal one, but learned that a biochemist at the University of Georgia emulsified the box of a popular cereal and separately ground up the cereal then fed one group of rats the box and another the cereal. The ones that ate the box thrived and the others did not. This speaks volumes about the quality of our processed foods.

I have seen parents get into the most embarrassing situations over their children's eating. An anxious parent will try and force the child to eat and naturally the child rebels. So the parent caves in and begins to offer tit bits of junk food to tempt the child into eating. Quickly the child learns that the one way in which she can express her independence and exercise some power over her anxious parents is to rebel. In this way a nasty cycle has been created of a fussy eater who holds the whole family to ransom and whose behaviour becomes erratic while nervous parents worry that the child is going to starve to death. My advice? Hang in there and simply offer a variety of high-quality foods. Have bowls of fruit available between meals and eventually your child will come round. Food consumption will vary enormously and seems to be tied into growth spurts. Remember never to use food as a bribe, a reward or as compensation. Not only can this result in obesity but it results in food not being about nourishment and pleasure.

Try and introduce most foods before the first birthday raw and liquidised and after that by all means introduce steamed and pureed vegetables, boiled and mashed potatoes, pre-soaked low-heated grains which are then liquidised and pulses. Young children are particularly fond of sprouted seeds once their teeth have come through and they are so easy to grow and fun to chew. Introduce grains one at a time as some children react poorly to wheat. Buckwheat, millet and rice are usually fine. Salads and vegetables don't seem to go down a bundle with many young children so it is a good idea to liquidise raw vegetables. One of my favourite recipes is the Spanish one for tomato soup, Gazpacho, which is easily made. I usually pour mine over a base of whole wheat liquidised breadcrumbs soaked in a little lemon juice and olive oil. So far I have not had any young children reject this adult version of a liquidised salad!

Snacks between meals can be healthy and include halva made with grape juice instead of sugar (available from health-food shops), home made ice-cream (freeze a banana and once frozen liquidise it in your blender at high speed) as well as fruit-juice ice lollies, corn popped in olive oil, dried unsulphured fruit, and homemade biscuits and cake.

If you do make biscuits and cakes at home try to use maple syrup, blackstrap unsulphured molasses, or honey – never sugar which could be the thin edge of the wedge. Some prepacked cereals are almost 50 per cent sugar as are carbonated drinks. It is now possible to buy carbonated drinks containing natural sweeteners from health-food shops, but I wouldn't recommend them too often because carbon dioxide is a waste gas and should not be forced down your child. Happily most children don't like ordinary coffee or tea which is just as well, but they do like chocolate which interferes with the calcium metabolism and damages the liver. It is also too high in copper which can contribute to the development of diabetes. Carob is a much better substitute. Most young children don't like strong spices, salt, black pepper, mustard, etc., which is a healthy attitude as they can be harsh irritants to the delicate lining of the digestive tract.

• ALLERGIES •

Unless you have been living on Mars you will already know that colouring, preservatives and flavouring are not good for a child and can lead to all sorts of behavioural problems as well as a damaged immune system. A bad reaction to a specific food can be the result of a baby or child not having the enzymes she needs to digest it (as with lactose intolerance), or it may be the result of a confused and sensitised digestive system which is has become accustomed to a diet of junk. Wheat and dairy products are the two most common allergens. Ironically your child might land up craving for a food that she is reacting badly to. Initially negative symptoms such as catarrh or behavioural changes can become hidden and replaced by a craving or positive addiction for the damaging food. If your child has an inordinate desire for a certain food you can suspect an allergy. Try taking her off it altogether for fourteen days and watch carefully for any behavioural changes or physical alterations. It is common for the child to get worse while the food to which she is allergic clears from the system. Then you can reintroduce it and observe the changes. Some children can occasionally cope with a little of the food to which they have an intolerance (although I would not recommend this).

It helps not to serve liquids with meals which simply dilute the digestive juices. The only exception to this is diluted vegetable juice, vegetable broths and herbal teas. The quality of the water you use is of particular importance. I have known many young children react particularly badly to the chlorine and fluoride in water.

Finally, bear in mind that food prepared and served with love in a happy peaceful environment is much more nutritious than even the best-quality food served in a battle-ground atmosphere. Food that is blessed has an higher auric energy than food that is fought over. Remember it is not what you eat but what you assimilate that counts and assimilation is enhanced if the whole family enjoy eating together or separately in a loving and positive environment.

• SUN AND AIR BATHING •

Sun and air bathing continue to be important for growing children. I remember as a child enjoying some exhilarating rain baths when I lived in the tropics of East Africa. It is a good and natural childish instinct to tear off all those clothes and run outside in a heavy tropical storm. Children tend to be discouraged from exposing their bodies to the elements and synthetic fabrics and shoes all take their toll with human health.

• SLEEP •

Children are best allowed to go to sleep at dusk and get up at dawn. Hours spent within a 12 foot (3.6 metres) radius of a television set will mean exposure to ELFs and may lead to disturbed sleep.

• EXERCISE •

Most children these days don't get enough exercise and obesity is an epidemic amongst them as a result. Exercise not only expands growing lungs, oxygenates the blood and develops the muscles but it helps digestion and appetite. Lazy couch-bound parents make for lazy lumpy children!

• SPIRITUALITY •

In my opinion your efforts to help develop emotional, intellectual and spiritual facilities in your child are even more important than feeding them good organic foods. For the first few years of your child's life her home is her whole world. It is utterly impossible to spoil your child with too much love. Unlimited and unconditional love will have an amazing affect on her future mental, moral and social development. Personality traits don't come automatically nor are they learned in school, rather they are instilled and implanted in your child's character during earliest childhood by your own positive examples and influences and by contacts within her immediate society. Use your own parental intuition, inspiration and spiritual insight as your guide and if your child can say to you as Thomas Jefferson did to his parents, 'The happiest moments of my life have been the few which I passed at home in the bosom of my family', you can rest assured you have done a wonderful job.

CHAPTER 8:

A-Z OF MINOR AILMENTS FOR BABIES AND TODDLERS

———

• BED WETTING •

Bed wetting is sometimes due to oxalic acid crystals in the kidneys or bladder causing irritation and other causes include eating too late, constipation, parasites and very often general nervousness.

Cut all stimulating foods out of the diet including spices, tea, coffee, fizzy drinks and refined foods and don't allow a late meal. Stop all liquids after five o'clock in the evening and before bed apply olive oil, gently warmed, massaged over the kidney area. Encourage your child to lie on her side. I've instructed some mothers to make a cloth ball and fasten it into the back of the pyjamas so that a child cannot turn over on to her back and this works quite well. If a child is thirsty before bed give her fresh fruit instead of liquids.

I have long used Dr Christopher's excellent bed-wetting formulation with great success. It is made from equal parts of finely powdered marshmallow root, black cohosh, parsley root, uva ursi, juniper berries, white pond lily, goldenseal, ginger, white poplar, sumach berries and yarrow. Give two size 2 capsules morning and evening with a cup of parsley tea which has been sweetened. If your child cannot swallow capsules mix the powdered herbs, a quarter of a teaspoon, into a little maple syrup.

CHICKEN POX

Follow the advice for Fever (see pages 152–4) and also bathe the skin externally with decoctions of yellow dock or goldenseal root in cases of severe itching. If she is slow in breaking out in spots give her a good warm bath.

COLDS

Think of a cold as a natural purification process and don't try to stop it. Any time a cold is discouraged and suppressed with chemical remedies it will drag on in one form or another for several months. A cold that is properly managed should last for two to three days at the most. Ideally a child should be encouraged to fast on fruit juice, potassium broth and herbal tea for two to three days but don't extend the fast beyond this time as it tends to prolong the cold.

Every child I have ever met who has been bought up naturally has a wonderful self-preservation instinct when ill and will naturally stop eating. It is only parents worried cajoling and entreaties to eat – certain that their baby is going to fade away without access to food on a regular basis – that distorts this natural instinct. You will notice that when animals are hurt they instinctively fast. This is because the body needs all its energy to heal, not to digest food, so a fast for a few days when fighting a streaming cold is strongly recommended. Do not extend the fasting beyond this time as it tends to prolong the cold but help the child with a diet full of onions, garlic and citrus fruits.

One of the most delicious and effective teas I have found for a cold is a decoction of ginger root, strained with plenty of honey and lemon added, a generous pinch of cayenne pepper and a crushed clove of garlic in each mug.

Hot mustard foot baths will decongest the head and, if the child can manage, a salt water douche into the nose using a nasal spray will open up and decongest the sinuses. Facial steam inhalations using Olbas oil are a helpful alternative. Composition Essence which is made up of equal parts of elderflowers, peppermint and yarrow can be stirred into hot water according to the instructions on the bottle (see Resources Directory) and sipped hot frequently.

COLD SORES

Apply neat tincture of golden seal or T-tree oil directly on to the cold sore and add plenty of fresh garlic to the diet. Internally administer equal parts of scullcap and golden seal in tincture form according to age. The dose for a child over eight is five drops hourly until the cold sore stops hurting and then five drops three times a day until it is cleared completely.

NB Cold sores are very infectious so don't encourage any kissing or passing the baby round the family while the child is infected. Be especially careful not to pass cold sores on to a child with eczema.

CONJUNCTIVITIS

> *If your child has an eye infection seek immediate medical advice before employing herbal treatments.*

If your baby has an eye infection suspect a plugged tear duct and massage the duct gently with golden seal tea. The causes of conjunctivitis (distinct reddening of the white part of the eye) may be due to external irritants or infections from bacteria or herpes. Conjunctivitis itself never causes persistent visual disturbance. Bathe the eye with a meticulously strained tea of golden seal, eyebright or raspberry leaf three or four times a day and introduce plenty of garlic to the diet (see above).

CONSTIPATION

A very high percentage of all diseases and malfunctions of children's bodies come from a congested intestinal tract and lack of co-ordination in the nerve and muscle function of the colon and bowel. I've treated many children who have inherited weaknesses in the colon so that they came out of the womb unable to have proper bowel movements. In an emergency I will administer enemas or use colonic irrigation but I aim to re-educate the bowel so that eventually it will function properly with the aid of nothing but a healthy diet.

I've already made it very clear that a diet of fruits, vegetables, nuts, grains, seeds and soya products (preferably taking at least half of these raw), promotes proper bowel function. The real culprits of constipation are foods that have a binding nature like meat, dairy products and highly refined foods, all of which have little or no life in them. Wheat flower, for example, makes an excellent wallpaper paste and white glue is a by-product of the dairy industry made from proteins in milk. The walls of Venice, which have been standing for hundreds of years, were originally made of dirt and eggs.

The improved circulation and lung capacity produced by vigorous exercise together with the strengthening of abdominal muscles all stimulate the peristaltic action of the bowel. Peristalsis is simply a wave-like movement by which waste matter travels through and eventually out of the colon. So exercise is a vital factor for good bowel health.

Emotions will drastically affect a child's ability to have a bowel movement. Fear is directly linked with constipation.

If a baby is not breast fed from birth she runs the risk of having very poor intestinal ecology. Even a young child's colon will hold nearly a pound of resident bacteria as indigenous flora. This is composed of three or four hundred different species of bacteria whose activities have wide-reaching affects on the metabolism, physiology and bio-chemistry and these micro organisms can be either indigenous or transient. Those that are indigenous colonise the intestinal tract by adhering to the gut lining; while those that are transient are ingested in food and drink on an on-going basis. Together they make up nearly 40 per cent of the whole weight of your child's faecal matter. Putrefactive bacteria take care of the decaying matter in the colon and thrive on a diet full of protein and fat which accelerates the output of undesirable metabolites like bile salts, urea, phenols and ammonia, all of which are potentially harmful, doubly so if a child is already constipated or has jaundice. A high population of bacterioids contributes to the development of degenerative diseases such as ultractive colitis, diverticulitis and haemorrhoids. Many people in the West have a ratio of 85 per cent of these potentially harmful bacteria to only 15 per cent of the beneficial bacteria which produce acids that, among other things, prevent the colonisation of fungus like candida albicans. Once the percentage is better balanced (and it should be ideally in the converse ratio) peristalsis is stimulated, flushing out toxic bacterial metabolites and waste products in the faeces and so checking putrefactive bacteria.

There are foods which directly promote benign intestinal flora including natural, raw, unsalted sauerkraut, miso soup and fermented grains, as well as garlic which is capable of destroying harmful bacteria while actively encouraging good bacteria. The most vicious destroyers of beneficial intestinal flora are antibiotics. The only way I would ever consider giving a child antibiotics is in a life-threatening situation. If your child has to have antibiotics also get some probiotics (see Resources Directory) and administer them according to instructions for at least six weeks afterwards to recolonise the good intestinal flora they will have destroyed.

Radiation of the abdomen, including X-rays, upsets the normal microbial balance of the colon, as does sudden violent changes in the weather and loud prolonged music above 72 decibels. Useful information if your child is a teenager! Stress also has a profound affect on intestinal ecology no matter what its source. Cumulatively, all of these reactions alter the intestinal habitat decreasing the micro-organic goodies and increasing the baddies.

Bowel movements are not something that are discussed in detail in most families and yet when you consider that later in life 60 per cent of all cancers shared by men and women are colon rectal cancers, this type of information given to a child early in life is both vital and invaluable.

Help your child to understand that having a bowel movement should be easy, comfortable and quick. Never discourage them when they feel the urge. They should be able to evacuate their bowel in less than two minutes and be finished without squeezing, straining or grunting. Every bowel movement should be soft and mushy like cottage cheese, slightly gaseous and should crumble and break as it reaches the water in the toilet. If it is well formed or any harder or dryer than this the child is constipated and this may lead to haemorrhoids later in life. A child ideally should have a bowel movement for every meal she eats.

The following suggestions will help to promote better bowel elimination. Begin with the gentler steps first.

1. Drink a minimum of one gallon of water, herbal teas or diluted juices every day. Dehydration of faecal matter is a major factor in chronic constipation. It is very hard for dried-up faecal matter to travel through the colon, and liquid simply hydrates it and makes peristalsis easier.
2. Cathartic fruit juices such as prune and fig have long been famous for their bowel-cleansing abilities, but apple juice is also quite effective, as is pear juice. Prune juice has the ability of drawing in waste through the colon wall from the surrounding bloodstream, so this is particularly recommended. Drink up to two quarts daily, preferably freshly juiced and well 'chewed', served at room temperature.
3. Mucilaginous herbs like phyllium seeds and flax seeds are capable of absorbing many times their natural weight in water and so bulk up in the colon and act like a soft sponge to push faecal matter through and

encourage peristalsis. Flax seeds are also rich in their own natural lubricating oil.

4. Ginger root greatly increases bowel activity. Administer it in the form of a delicious ginger root decoction with plenty of honey and lemon added and give this liberally as needed.

5. Garlic, as previously mentioned, actively encourages the growth of benign flora in the colon and acts as an antiseptic, destroying unfriendly bacteria. Garlic is also one of the few herbs that not only kills intestinal parasites but also actively expels them.

6. Cascara sagrada bark, senna pods and/or leaves, and aloes are all rich in emodin. Emodin has a direct action on the smooth muscle of the large intestine, stimulating it and encouraging it to move. Aloes are generally twice as strong as cascara sagrada. The two best known are cape aloes and curacao aloes, and these are much more powerful than aloe vera. The juice of aloe vera or its gel are commonly available in health-food shops and have much milder properties than either cape or curacao aloes in their whole form.

The formulations on page 97 and 99 are also very helpful and a child, particularly one who's heavily constipated and in pain, will almost always take these formulations willingly when mixed with a little maple syrup, date syrup or molasses. I've had some parents who put this mixture inside a date which can then be chewed and swallowed. I would only graduate to giving these formulas to a child after having gone through the previously listed steps without success.

COUGHS

Happily most babies don't get infections, but if a baby does go down with a cough or cold it can quickly turn into pneumonia so keep a very close and careful eye on your baby. If she is only one or two months old and develops irregular breathing, coughing and looks limp and pale do consult a doctor straight away because it could mean she has pneumonia, even if there is no fever. If your child is exposed to other people's colds and coughs remember garlic is a great antibiotic and echinacea builds the immune system while fighting viruses. These are not too difficult to get down young children but a baby can be treated by putting a few drops of echinacea tincture directly on to your nipple if you are breast feeding and allowing the child to suck. You can use garlic oil for a tiny baby in the same way. If the child is older than three months, you can feed very finely minced garlic mixed with a little liquid acidophilus or boiled water to the baby directly off a teaspoon, but because it tastes so hot it needs to be immediately subdued afterwards by a good nursing session. If the baby is older I have found tincture of plantain (10 drops in water is needed) or garlic or onion syrup (one teaspoon as often as needed) extremely affective. Remember a cough is simply natures way of clearing an infection in the bronchial passages whereby bacteria is being immobilised and thereby protecting the lungs from damage. A cough should never, for this reason, be suppressed. To make onion or garlic syrup cover several finely sliced onions or three to four bulbs of sliced and peeled garlic with Manukau honey. This superb honey from New Zealand has been shown to kill many strains of bacteria and is the one I employ for all medicinal use. Keep on a low heat at about 54°C (130°F) for several hours, and then strain and cool it. Encourage the child to hold the syrup in the mouth and let it trickle slowly down the throat. To ease the pain of coughing rub the chest with a little olbas oil or apply a ginger compress. If the cough is one of those irritating ones that goes on for some days, encourage the child to sip a decoction of equal parts of wild cherry bark, aniseed and wild lettuce liberally laced with Manukau honey. Dispense as often as needed and certainly every two hours.

> *If any cough lasts more than a week, you must seek professional help as it may need further investigation.*

CRADLECAP

This is a yellow deposit as the scalp of babies, caused by seborrhoea. Ensure that your baby is getting plenty of calcium tea (see page 102). Saturate the head every night in organic olive oil with a few drops of added rosemary or lavender oil and in the morning massage the loosened crusts off. These will come away with a soft baby brush or a clean finger nail but don't be tempted to pick off crusts that are not loose as this may cause bleeding and subsequent infection of the scalp.

After using a natural soap (see Resources Directory) to shampoo, rinse with an infusion of burdock afterwards. Don't be tempted to wash your child's hair too frequently as this will merely aggravate sebum secretion which is the cause of the problem in the first place. This condition can actually last until the child is three, but it presents no health problems. Most mothers like to remove it simply because they don't like the look of it.

CROUP

Give the child a hot mustard foot bath followed by a catnip tea enema if possible. Rub the chest with olbas oil or deep heat oil (see Resources Directory) and administer equal parts of catnip and peppermint tea with a few drops of tincture of lobelia in it often.

DIARRHOEA

Diarrhoea is caused by a substance irritating the colon so badly that peristalsis goes into overdrive in an attempt to expel it.

> *Chronic diarrhoea which goes on for several days or recurs persistently obviously needs professional help and any diarrhoea in infancy which does not clear up within twenty-four hours needs immediate and urgent medical attention.*

Slippery elm gruel is excellent for a tiny baby with diarrhoea. Always ensure that you keep the bottom really well wiped to prevent soreness. In older children oatmeal porridge simply prepared with water can be both soothing and helpful, and probiotics specifically designed for children will encourage the correct ecology of the colon.

EARACHE

> *Ears are very delicate, sensitive and complex organs. They can be damaged easily by neglect or inappropriate treatment. If you are in any doubt at all about the cause of an earache in your baby or toddler consult your doctor.*

If the earache is the result of a chill, apply a raw grated onion poultice over the back and sides of the neck, securing it with a cotton bandage. Put a few drops of mullein or garlic oil into both ears, even if the earache is only in one ear, and plug with cotton wool.

A hot foot bath may help the pain of earache as will any source of heat locally applied; for example, lying on a hot water bottle that is well wrapped in a towel.

In an emergency if no herbs are available use diluted lemon juice, a teaspoon to a cup of tepid water, dripped into both ears. In all instances you can rub the lymph glands below the ears with the same preparations as you have used internally. Attend to your own diet if you are breast feeding because you may be taking too many dairy products or eating something which is creating an allergy in your baby.

FEVERS

> *All fevers should be seen by your GP and any usage of herbs discussed with him or her.*

I place chicken pox, measles, mumps, scarlet fever and whooping cough all under the general heading of fevers because these feverish ailments of childhood require similar treatment. First let me explain to you what a fever is and how, properly managed, it can be one of natures most efficient healing tools. When too much mucus, toxic waste, or synthetic drugs accumulate within the body its natural reaction is to unload this material before it reaches a high enough level to actually endanger the body and cause death. The body then reacts with colds and other childhood diseases and the first indication of disease is usually a fever. Aim to assist a fever in your child to rebuild a malfunctioning area with cleaning and feeding processes. During the fever the body is drawing healing aids from itself (provided of course there are some there) and discarding and burning up unwanted materials. Trying to stop a fever artificially with synthetic drugs, as many frightened parents do, is tantamount to bailing out a sinking boat without plugging up the bung hole.

The majority of fevers are caused by viral or bacterial infections and are part of the body's own immune response to invasion. Whenever an infection develops a child responds by creating new leucocytes (white blood cells) and in an emergency their passage around the body accelerates to fight the baddies. In the process pyrogens are released specifically to raise body temperature and make this cleansing process more efficient. For every degree your child's temperature increases it speeds their activity by ten times so that by the time your child has a temperature of 104°F the leucocytes are working sixty-four times faster than normal. Children tend to get astonishingly high temperatures very quickly simply because they are so full of vitality their healing processes are extremely efficient and very intense. Our ageing bodies slow down and tend to loose this rapid healing ability.

So a temperature during a fever, properly managed, is to be encouraged. To take your child's temperature the safest way is to place a thermometer under the armpit.

In new-born babies it's important to get a doctor's advice with fever because there could be a chance of infection having developed as the result of foetal monitoring during birth or some forced obstetric procedure. It is extremely unusual for a new-born to develop a fever during a natural birthing process which is properly managed. Sometimes children can become feverish as a result of being over-dressed, exposed to too much sun, over excited or a tooth breaking through. If you suspect they've swallowed a poisonous substance you need to seek immediate medical help.

The rule for fever is: dry fever is dangerous but wet fever heals. So make sure your child's body remains full of fluid. I've known some babies not to take anything when they are sick but most will accept breast milk, so make sure your breast milk is running at its most voluminous by drinking plenty of blessed thistle or marsh-mallow root tea and allow the baby to nurse as long and as often as she wants to. If she refuses to take anything run a nice deep warm bath with added infusions of catnip ginger or camomile tea and get in with the baby, topping up with more hot water as necessary and sponging both of you off with cold water at the end. Babies sweat and rehydrate gratifyingly quickly with this treatment. This is a good idea even if babies are nursing.

Apart from rehydration the next most important thing to do is check their bowels and see if your baby or child is constipated. If a child is capable of swallowing anything offer a herbal tea made of three parts of turkey rhubarb, two parts comfrey root and one part liquorice root (which is a nice sweetener) and give one cup three times a day for children who are twelve years old and over, half a cup three times a day for eight to twelve year olds and reduced amounts proportionately for younger children according to age.

The third most important step is to keep sponging your child down constantly with a mixture of half apple cider vinegar and half water (which will ensure that the pH balance of the skin is maintained). Make sure this water is used lukewarm and follow the sponging process every hour. This will keep the temperature within a reasonable range. Abdominal compresses are also very useful as they stimulate the liver and activate the circulation so speeding up the body's natural detoxification process. Make sure your child is in a warm, shaded and well ventilated room. Dip a piece of white cotton into cold water. It should be wide enough to wrap around the whole body from beneath the armpits to the groin. Wrap it closely around the skin and secure it with safety pins then put on a thick dry cotton towel and slip the child into a warmed bed with hot water bottles and a pair of thick bed socks made from cotton or wool. Keep it on for half an hour, although it may be left on all night if the child is sleeping. This can be repeated several times a day, depending on the level of your child's temperature.

Fourthly, never force your child to eat but do encourage plenty of liquids, particularly hot potassium broth, freshly pressed and diluted juices and purified water. The juices can be anything that the child particularly enjoys. Also administer diaphoretic teas (that is herbal teas that make a child sweat). Babies will usually take catnip, camomile or elderflower tea without complaint and young children also enjoy peppermint and ginger teas. If a baby will not take any of these teas you can always administer them sweetened with a little maple syrup through an eye dropper. Babies can be given several dropperfuls every few hours and children may drink as much as desired. If breast feeding by all means drink these teas yourself so the baby will get the benefit of them.

There is an old adage that 'old people and children fast badly'. I've noticed that this tends to be true, so when a child's appetite comes back spontaneously don't insist on an over-long fast. Offer fresh fruits, if necessary liquidised into smoothies, to break a fast, and remember a child in bed is usually a bored child so this is the time for story telling and planning exciting projects for the future as well as looking at new books and puzzles. If your child is restless and can't sleep, give equal parts of catnip, peppermint and spearmint tea sweetened with maple syrup before bed.

INDIGESTION

Children usually only suffer from indigestion as the result of bad eating habits or eating in an atmosphere charged with distress. To my mind it is one of the easiest complaints to rectify without having to resort to herbal medicine provided eating habits are altered and the food-combining rules are followed. Ensure that meals are **always eaten** in a calm, quiet atmosphere at a leisurely pace.

1. Ensure your child chews properly and thoroughly. Cutting down on talking and playing quiet music will enable the child to concentrate on this.
2. Do not offer any liquid with the meals unless it is herbal tea, freshly pressed vegetable juice or potassium broth. If soup is being taken as part of a meal leave a fifteen-minute gap before offering the rest of the food.
3. Avoid salt, spicy foods, sugar, tea, coffee, fizzy drinks, refined carbohydrates (especially fried food) and anything else which you suspect may act as a gastric irritant for your child.
4. Do not offer excessively hot or ice-cold foods.
5. **Never offer a child any food to eat if they are distressed**. If the child tells you she is really hungry, offer a glass of freshly pressed vegetable juice at room temperature or a cup of potassium broth until she has completely calmed down.
6. **Never force a child to eat, particularly if they are ill**.
7. No arguments at the table!
8. If food is eaten too soon after a previous meal, the natural pace of the digestive process will be disrupted so allow two hours respite after a fruit meal and three hours after a vegetable one.
9. If none of this helps investigate the possibility of an intolerance to dairy products or wheat or the presence of candidiasis with a professional herbalist. Distortion of the thoracic vertebrae can also upset the stomach and needs osteopathic help.

Note that milk can actually increase hydrochloric acid secretion and make symptoms far worse so don't offer the child milk or milk shakes.

Serve this tea made of equal parts of peppermint, fennel and ginger with meals. Sweeten it with plenty of honey. It tastes delicious. Allow the child to sip as much of this as desired.

INFANTILE ECZEMA

When the kidneys and liver can't cope with toxic waste and the lungs are an inappropriate avenue for them, the one remaining organ that the body can employ to excrete poisons is the skin. Skin problems lumped under the general heading of eczema or dermatitis are the result. A distressed skin is the body's outward manifestation of an excretory overload, so it is essential, if you observe a skin problem in your child, to ensure the other channels of elimination are working properly, that is the kidneys, the liver, the lungs, the bowel and the lymphatic system. Check the body isn't being overloaded with external poisons such as chemicals or additives that it cannot cope with. Eczema is now a common complaint among European children and is exacerbated, in my opinion, by potent pharmaceuticals which mask but do not solve the problem.

It has been proven, as long ago as 1936, that the general instance of infantile eczema is 'lowest in breast-fed infants. In the partially breast-fed it is twice as frequent as in the breast-fed, and in the artificially-fed infants, seven times as great'. Undoubtedly cows' milk is the most common allergy-causing food but interestingly, feeding cows' milk in early infancy exacerbates gluten intolerance later in life. Long years of clinical practice lead me to concur with the fact that dairy products and wheat are major causes of infantile eczema. However, sometimes eczema can be caused by reaction to certain materials, particularly synthetic fabrics, as well as to toxins in the air and environment. Babies reared in an over warm house where the air is particularly dry can often get chronically itchy skin. Some babies and children need extra linoleic acid or B vitamins. The former is available in copious quantities in evening primrose and borage flower oil and the latter in nutritional yeast. Very occasionally I have found that a heavily spiced diet can cause eczema in certain susceptible children and I have treated several Indian children whose eczema was partly exacerbated by their highly spiced diet.

The first thing to observe is not to use any soap while washing and if the chlorine in the water irritates the skin, as it does many children, neutralise it with a teaspoon of sodium thiosulphate in each bath, running the bath with the window open. This is available from chemists. A bag full of oatmeal can be left soaking in the water and used instead of soap. Pinhead oatmeal tied in a muslin bag with a rubber band works very effectively for this purpose.

Ensure that the baby or child's bowels are working properly and that the diet, whether it be through the breast milk of the mother or straight off the plate, is at its best. I have had a great deal of success with tincture of heartsease administered internally, the dose dependent upon age.

Maurice Messegue, the famous French herbalist, used the following hand and foot baths which he claimed were 98 per cent successful. Here is his formulation.

Boil up a quart of water in anything but aluminium or copper and allow it to cool until lukewarm, and drop in a handful of each of the following herbs: artichoke leaves, elecampane flowers and leaves, fresh celandine leaves (although if the season is wrong dried will do), chicory root, broom flowers, lavender flowers and nettle leaves (preferably fresh, but dried will do). Allow the mixture, having stirred it in well with a wooden spoon, to soak for four to five hours. Strain and pour this into a clean bottle for storage until it needs to be used. This mixture can be kept in the fridge for up to eight days without deteriorating.

Use this in an eight-minute foot bath each morning before breakfast and an eight-minute hand bath in the evening before dinner. Hand and foot baths are easily adapted to and often very much enjoyed by young children. Make the bath in the following way. Boil two quarts of water and let it stand for five minutes. Add half a pint (300 ml) of the previously prepared herbal mixture to two quarts (2 litres) of boiled water. Encourage the child to take a foot or hand bath as hot as they can manage. This mixture may be reused the same day, and simply warmed up. Then begin again.

Marigold, evening primrose or borage oil massaged into dry scaly eczema externally is very effective, as is chickweed or comfrey ointment. A raw cucumber juice poultice can be very soothing applied to an itchy sore skin as can aloe vera fresh gel (see Resources Directory). Exposure to a little natural light is also extremely helpful, as is the wearing of 100 per cent natural undyed cotton.

IMPETIGO

This is a very infectious skin disease caused by a bacterial infection which manifests itself by producing pus-filled itching lesions. These then burst and crust over; the golden crusts appear mainly on the face, hands and knees. Clean out the bloodstream with anti-bacterial herbs like echinacea, garlic or golden seal and wipe the area down with equal parts of T-tree oil and castor oil. Ensure that there is plenty of raw garlic in the diet which, as it is not to every child's taste, can be used as part of the filling in a baked potato or in garlic bread. Also ensure plenty of raw freshly pressed carrot juice, which is high in vitamin A, is taken.

MEASLES

If the child is slow in breaking out in a fever (see pages 5, 152–4) give them a good hot bath. Make sure the room is kept dark so that eyes do not become irritated. If they do become sore bathe them with an infusion, meticulously strained, of equal parts of eyebright, raspberry and golden seal. If the skin is sore follow the instructions for chicken pox.

MUMPS

In addition to following the fever advice (see pages 5, 152–4) apply a poultice of three parts mullein and one part lobelia herb around the neck and swollen area covering with plastic and a cloth or towel over the plastic to prevent leaking on to the bed. Renew the poultice every half hour for the first day and, if comfortable, leave it on all night. Also administer one cup of the tea in the same proportions (more or less according to age) three or more times a day.

NAPPY RASH

So called primitive tribes who don't use nappies have babies which, unsurprisingly, seldom suffer from this problem. When I was a little girl in Kenya I would observe mothers simply cleaning themselves off when the baby urinated and most of them, because they wore the child strapped to their back or chests every waking moment, developed such intuition and harmony with the baby that they understood exactly when the child needed to urinate and could easily swing the child off their bodies out of their sling, holding them away from them and allowing them to urinate so that the soiling of themselves was avoided. So the obvious first step to avoid nappy rash is to allow sunshine and air to a baby's bottom as often as possible. Keeping your baby clean and waterproof after each bowel movement is essential. The best mixture for this is 90 per cent Johoba oil mixed with 10 per cent T-tree oil. Jojoba is actually more of a wax than an oil and is extremely waterproof but easily absorbed, while T-tree oil is antifungal, antiviral and antibacterial.

If the rash is the result of a yeast infection you need to cut out all forms of sugar from your diet if you are breast feeding (see pages 96–97) and from your baby's diet if she is eating anything. Use garlic oil over the rash and make sure your baby or toddler is given appropriate probiotics (see Resources Directory). Please avoid any petrol-based products such as mineral oil on the baby's skin as well as talcum powder which is known to cause cancer.

PRICKLY HEAT

The first step is to keep your baby cool because prickly heat generally happens as the result of hot sticky weather. Ensure that your baby is wearing the minimum amount of natural fabrics in a well-ventilated area. When bathing use corn starch afterwards as a powder having first bathed the skin with a teaspoon of baking soda diluted in a cup of water dabbed on with a pure cotton cloth. Vitamin C is a very effective treatment for prickly heat. Children over eight can take 500 mg a day, those under eight 250 mgs and babies can be given 25 mg dissolved in pure water and fed with a dropper.

STYES

Styes are usually a symptom that a child is extremely run down and rubbing it with a piece of raw potato, preferably organic, will help to calm the unbearable itchiness. Bathe the eyes regularly with a meticulously strained decoction of golden seal and if the child will allow it, apply a warm compress of golden seal over a closed eyelid for twenty minutes. Eyesight problems are helped by a diet which is as healthy as possible, i.e. high in raw foods and totally vegan.

SUNBURN

Ideally tender babies skin should not be exposed to the sun for more than ten minutes at a time and if a child sunbathes regularly she will not burn herself. A good anti-sunburn lotion to rub on before sunbathing is a teaspoon of apple cider vinegar in half a cup of olive oil. Then dampen the piece of cotton wool, wringing out most of the moisture, dip this into the oil and rub it evenly over the skin.

In cases of severe sunburn, first lie the child in a cold bath until she feels chilled and then pat dry very gently and apply the following paste. Equal parts of liquid organic honey and vitamin E oil blended with pulverised fresh or dried comfrey leaf so it is the consistency of a thick, heavy but spreadable paste. Apply it half an inch thick (1.25 cm) or more over the entire area that's been burned and cover with gauze, bandaging lightly. Observe the area regularly and if the paste becomes absorbed simply apply more on top. **Do not remove the original**, just add more as needed. This paste can be kept in the refrigerator in a screw-top jar for any type of burn on hand.

For travelling, aloe vera sprays and gels are also very useful (see Resources Directory).

TEETHING

Babies who develop fever, rashes, vomiting and irritability while teething are often short of assimilable calcium so should be fed calcium tea. If a fever does develop contact your GP and consult a medical herbalist if you wish to. Allowing the baby to chew on a piece of marshmallow root (hydrated if you can only get it dried) can be very helpful or alternatively on crushed ice put into a piece of gauze. Maple syrup mixed with a few drops of camomile oil rubbed into the gums can also be helpful, as can equal parts of catnip and fennel tincture massaged directly into the gums. Oil of cloves definitely numbs toothache but needs to be sweetened a little before being massaged in as its taste is too strong for babies. Gently massaging the babies fingers and toes which are roughly equivalent to the acupressure areas for the head can ease the pain too.

TONSILS

Tonsils have now been acknowledged by the medical profession to be a valuable part of the immune system and are best left in place if at all possible. If a child gets tonsillitis make sure that all the eliminative channels are opening and working properly, particularly the lymphatic system. Gargle with five drops of T-tree oil, myrrh, echinacea, or golden seal in half a tumbler of water frequently. Echinacea is particularly soothing if sprayed directly into the throat and certainly helps with pain. Apply a poultice externally of equal parts of mullein and lobelia. If the tonsillitis is chronic, that is it recurs, mix equal parts of thuja tincture and glycerine and paint them directly on to the tonsils with a camel-hair brush while including plenty of fresh garlic in the diet. A three-day fast on fruit juices is highly recommended.

TOOTHACHE

Before using herbs first consult your dentist as soon as possible. Make sure there is no impacted food around the aching tooth by using dental floss and apply an ice pack against the jaw on the infected side. Pack any visible cavity with a piece of crushed garlic or pour a small amount of oil of cloves into it. Rub ice over the web of the finger between the thumb and the index finger on the same side of the body as the pain is because this is the acupressure point used to relieve toothache.

Please do not let your child use a fluoridated toothpaste. High levels of fluoride are believed to be associated with cancer, genetic disorders, brittle bones and mottled teeth. The problem is that most of us consume too much fluoride from natural sources such as food and drink, as well as being exposed to artificial sources like insecticides, anaesthetics and preservatives. Children can only excrete about a third of the fluoride they swallow and even very low levels of fluoride inhibit the ability of leucocytes (infection-fighting white blood cells) to migrate, which means fluoride depresses the immune system.

Children's spitting reflexes to the age of three are very poor and they swallow most of the toothpaste they use.

URINARY INFECTIONS

Happily inflammation of the bladder is rare among children. Common symptoms include pain and burning on urination. Cloudy, sour smelling, or bloody urination, backache, chills and quite high fevers are all indications. Make sure your child is not wearing clothes washed by bleaches and detergents next to the skin and avoid fabric coloured by chemical dyes in their underwear. Do not let her wash with soap, particularly around the genital area. Running water will do just as well. Give her a cup of cranberry juice, preferably unsweetened, morning and evening with two drops of T-tree oil added to each cup, and encourage her to drink plenty of potassium broth. If she complains of soreness use a warm compress of fennel oil, ten drops diluted in enough water to moisten the compress, over the bladder and wrap her up well, keeping the rest of the body warm.

VOMITING

A small baby will dehydrate very quickly so you must be careful to maintain hydration if she vomits. One of the easiest ways to do this is simply to hold your baby in the bath while ensuring the room is kept very warm. Add a strong infusion of strained camomile tea to the water to ensure nourishment and relaxation. Then take the baby out of the bath and sponge her down with a cool mixture of half water and half apple cider vinegar. Pat her dry and massage her with olive oil thoroughly all over. One or two drops of tincture of lobelia placed directly into the baby's mouth can relax the tense muscles that cause vomiting. Some mothers have told me that my suggestion of using a thin gruel of slippery elm stays down when nothing else will. Once the vomiting has subsided feed the baby the following mixture by the teaspoonful: one teaspoon of freshly squeezed lemon juice, one teaspoon of organic maple syrup, a pinch of sea salt, all mixed into one cup of warm purified water. Similar to the electrolyte drinks that are sold commercially this is an excellent mixture to give after vomiting or diarrhoea to restore a child's strength.

WHOOPING COUGH

Part of the overall symptoms of whooping cough is a rapid accumulation of mucus in the throat which causes choking and needs to be eliminated as fast as possible. To cut the phlegm use a decoction of bayberry or oak bark as a gargle. It is fine to swallow this after gargling. Use a crushed clove of fresh garlic with half a teaspoon of cayenne pepper and a liberal lacing of honey in hot water and encourage the child to sip this every few minutes to clear the throat. A half teaspoon more of oil of garlic taken straight off the spoon is another alternative. Garlic oil can also be massaged into the throat, chest and back to give relief. Dr Shook's formulation specifically for whooping cough is excellent. Put two ounces of marshmallow root and two ounces of thyme into a quart of purified water and bring the herbs slowly to a simmer, continuing to do so until the mixture is reduced to one pint. Strain and add two pounds of honey. Dissolve thoroughly by stirring and then simmer for a further five minutes. If any scum rises to the surface skim it off. Cool and bottle keeping in a cold place. For children under four administer one teaspoon as often as needed for the cough. Older children may take three teaspoons at a time. This works very well for paroxysmal whooping cough bringing speedy relief. If used persistently it will eliminate the cough quickly and effectively. In addition to the treatment for fever encourage the child to gargle with a few drops of tincture of myrrh or golden seal in warm water, spitting the gargle out afterwards. Use oil from vitamin E capsules topically over any rash or sore area.

WORMS

This seems to be one of the topics that really gets parents going, as few of them are willing to believe that spanking clean children can get infested with worms. In truth pin worms, tape worms and round worms are quite common. Less common are hook worms and worms that arrive as the result of eating unclean pork. Symptoms of infestation include restlessness at night, picking the nose, gritting the teeth, itching around the anus and a dry cough. Worms can, in children, cause spasms, fits or convulsions. They come as the result of poor diet, poor hygiene and constipation. Simply trying to rid the body of worms is like killing flies and leaving behind rubbish (which has attracted them) in the same foul conditions. The root cause needs to be dealt with.

The first thing to do is start feeding the child a really good wholefood vegan diet together with plenty of freshly pressed juices, potassium broth and purified water. The most important step is to use the formula on page 162 to encourage a clean and healthy bowel and ensure that your child has a bowel movement for every meal eaten. This formulation can be administered by stirring it into a little maple syrup or honey if the child is too young to swallow capsules.

An infusion made of pumpkin seeds, preferably fresh, should be taken daily. Try and get your child to drink at least two cups of this. Fresh pumpkin seeds ground up and stirred into soup or cereal are also very helpful. Garlic, particularly fresh, is an excellent prophylactic for discouraging worms so include plenty of it in the diet. Other foods that discourage worms include onion, sage, mint, thyme and organic apple cider vinegar.

As far as children are concerned thread worms are by far the most common. Keep your child's fingernails very short and clean as these worms cause anal itching encouraging the child to scratch, so eggs then get into the fingernails and thus, by a circular route, into the child's mouth. They can also infect other children if foods are shared by hand. Fortunately the life cycle of these particular worms is only about sixteen days so, as long as you can prevent reinfection, you are winning. Often worms will creep from the anus to around the genital area. This can be prevented by massaging the whole area at night with garlic oil.

Antiparasitic formula

Equal parts of wormwood, black walnut, garlic, lobelia, burdock. Buy the herbs finely powdered and sieve well together. Give your child half a teaspoon of the powder mixed into unsulphured blackstrap molasses or maple syrup morning and evening for three days. On the fourth day give one cup of three parts of senna tea and one part of peppermint tea. Wait for two days and repeat the cycle. Do this two more times.

CHAPTER 9:

HERBAL FIRST AID FOR BABIES AND TODDLERS

———

The damage that toddlers can do to themselves can be quite horrifying for the unsuspecting and uninitiated parent and you owe it to yourself to have a well-stocked first-aid cabinet at home and a first-aid travel bag at the ready too in case of an emergency. This chapter is not designed to qualify anyone in first aid as it does not contain detailed instructions on bandaging, splinting, suturing or setting broken bones, but all of these useful skills can be learned at a first-aid class and I would advise you to enrol at least one member of your family in such a class. Most parents are terrified at the thought of an accident happening to their child and wouldn't know how to cope if one did, but by learning the most effective way in which to respond to any such accident you will quickly lose these terrors. Attendance at a first-aid course is the first step to doing this.

There are two particular situations where speedy action in dealing with the accident is especially vital. That is when a child has stopped breathing due to choking, electrical shock or drowning, or when a child is bleeding severely due to a large cut or puncture wound. If breathing has stopped, resuscitation should begin within minutes – this type of resuscitation is taught in first-aid classes. If a child is bleeding severely ensure that there are no foreign objects in the wound and then apply firm pressure. Raise and support the injured limb. Very serious bleeding from a major artery will require the use of a tourniquet which should be applied if you have a choice by someone properly trained in first-aid. Improperly used a tourniquet can result in blood vessel and nerve damage.

• BASIC ITEMS FOR YOUR FIRST-AID CABINET •

Ensure that your first-aid kit contains scissors, a thermometer, safety pins, tweezers, cotton wool, sterile eye pads, crêpe bandages, absorbent dressing, sterile gauze dressings, a small pack of paper tissues, perforated plasters, stretchy plasters and butterfly plasters.

• LIST OF ESSENTIAL HERBAL PREPARATIONS FOR A FIRST-AID CABINET •

Have a small supply of each of the following herbs in their dried and powdered form:

Cayenne
Slippery Elm
Comfrey
Charcoal (in powder or tablet form)
Intestinal Corrective No 3
Intestinal Corrective No 1 or 2 (capsule form decanted and clearly labelled in a self-sealed plastic bag).

Include the following tinctures:

Arnica
Cayenne
Echinacea
Golden seal
Plantain
Ginger

Include the following essential oils:

Lavender
Rosemary
T-Tree
St John's Wort
Cloves

Ensure you have a bottle of Rescue Remedy, Rescue Remedy cream, comfrey ointment and marigold cream. A small bottle of syrup of ipecacuana, some vitamin E oil in capsule form, a small jar of organic runny honey, a bulb of fresh garlic, a bottle of witchhazel, a bottle of Composition Essence, some Olbas oil, the tincture for insomnia, and a tincture for indigestion. Put any oils and tinctures in small one fluid ounce (30 ml) brown glass bottles with small droppers.

BLEEDING
Haemorrhage

> *If you have any suspicions of internal haemorrhage get the child to a doctor immediately.*

To stop an internal haemorrhage mix half a teaspoon of cayenne pepper in an eighth of a glass of warm water and get the child to drink it. Surprisingly, it doesn't taste hot if done in this way. Externally you can apply cayenne directly to a wound but do check that the wound is clean first. It is rich in vitamin A and so acts as an excellent disinfectant.

Nosebleed

For internal treatment see above and also encourage the child to sniff up a pinch of oak bark powder into each nostril. Apply ice to the back of the neck. If your child has frequent nosebleeds she may be calcium deficient so start feeding her the calcium tea.

• BURNS •

For first-degree burns (that is burns that affect the outer skin only causing redness, dryness, blistering and mild swelling) immerse the burn **immediately** in cold running water or rub it with ice cubes until all the pain has gone. This rapid response will stop blisters and modify any tissue damage. If the burn is extremely mild, cut the juicy leaf off an aloe vera plant, open it and apply the gelatinous contents directly to the burn. Alternatively, soak a piece of gauze in aloe vera juice and wrap it around the burn. Lavender oil, comfrey ointment, St John's Wort oil, marigold cream or the contents of vitamin E oil capsules are also helpful. Be aware that if you are using St John's Wort oil externally the burn should not be exposed to sunlight as it can cause skin discolouration.

For second-degree burns which involve the lower skin layers and may produce mottling, blisters or swelling, follow the same initial hydrotherapy then spread the vitamin E oil over the burn (use the contents of several capsules if the area is large). This will protect the skin while you prepare a paste of equal parts of powdered comfrey, runny organic honey and vitamin E oil. Now spread this evenly over the burn and **leave it on**. Do not attempt to peel it off. Simply add more as the skin absorbs it covering with gauze and a bandage. Continue to do this for a few days until all pain and swelling has subsided. If for any reason you do have to remove it (and try to avoid this) soak it off with a warm decoction of golden seal. Keep the burn out of the sun and as soon as the skin is strong enough, skin brush daily. Meanwhile ensure your child drinks plenty of carrot juice to accelerate the healing of the burn.

Acid burns

For acid burns flush the area immediately with one pint (600 mls) of cold water in which you have stirred a teaspoon of bicarbonate of soda. Apply poultices of ice-cold witchhazel, preferably non alcoholic, until the pain subsides and then smear with copious amounts of vitamin E oil, replenishing this every hour.

Third-degree burns

Third-degree burns which involve the full thickness of the skin require **immediate medical supervision** as these injuries can lead to severe loss of fluids and electrolytes, and shock and death are even possible. Powdered comfrey root stirred into juice and taken internally will accelerate the healing. On your way into hospital continue to soak the area in ice-cold water.

• TONGUE BURNS •

If a child burns her tongue sprinkle a few grains of sugar on it, and repeat this as often as necessary.

Burns from raw chillies or other blistering plant substances

If a child gets a plant rubbed on to their skin by accident that blisters, apply milk immediately and keep patting it on until the pain is soothed.

BRUISES

Apply an ice-cold compress of witchhazel to the bruise on a piece of gauze liberally sprinkled with tincture of arnica. Ice packs are useful and I keep cubes of frozen non-alcoholic witchhazel in my deep freezer which is an incredibly effective way to use this herb on bruises.

If a child bruises easily she may be short of vitamin C and it's complexes including hesperidin present in the white pith of citrus fruit.

CHILBLAINS

Unbroken chilblains

Provided the chilblains are not broken, hot mustard foot baths followed by cold dips are very helpful. Use one tablespoon of mustard powder to a bucket of hot water, so that the soak reaches to the knee. Repeat this hot/cold treatment eight times and repeat daily.

Alternatively, mix equal parts of cayenne pepper and corn starch and sprinkle this into your child's socks. A simpler method is snow walking. Encourage your child to walk barefoot on an even stretch of snow for ten seconds, gradually increasing to two or three minutes longer. When she does this she must always go outside well wrapped up and warmed up first except for the feet. Dry her feet by rubbing them well with your hands, not with a towel, and pop her into bed.

Sprouted buckwheat made into a porridge will assist the circulation by making the arteries more elastic.

Nelson's chilblain ointment is excellent if the chilblains are not broken.

Broken chilblains

If chilblains are broken, soak them in a warm infusion of dried marigold flowers then cover them with a poultice of the strained-out petals securing this in place with a bandage. Leave the poultice on the skin overnight and repeat the procedure until healed. Once the skin is healed apply marigold ointment until the redness has completely disappeared.

CUTS & MINOR WOUNDS

If the wound is bleeding copiously place it in ice-cold water or apply cayenne pepper directly. Both will arrest the bleeding and reduce inflammation. Now ensure the cut is absolutely clean. Proper cleansing is vital to help the wound heal easily and to prevent infection. Do ensure the wound is not so deep that it needs emergency micro-surgery. You may consider a cut deep enough if it goes through the skin and is long enough so that the sides of the cut separate and do not stay together. When a cut is this deep you will see shiny connective tissue or yellow globules of fat in the wound. If you are in any doubt about this go to your emergency accident unit and have it checked out. Having cleansed the wound properly to ensure-rapid healing and prevent infection apply neat T-tree or thyme oil. Both of them sting like crazy but they will stop any infection. A poultice of powdered comfrey mixed with a little honey will accelerate the healing or, if the cut is very superficial, use comfrey ointment.

If a large flap of skin is cut off, such as a finger tip, pressure should be applied to the cut to stop the bleeding. The piece of skin should then be put into ice-cold water or salt water, half a teaspoon of salt to two pints (1.2 litres) of water and taken along to the doctor. Generally it is possible to stitch the flap back on. However on two occasions I have used my own anti-infective tincture (see Resources Directory) followed by a poultice of wheatgerm oil, powdered comfrey and honey and healed such wounds without any scarring at all.

If the bleeding is copious and difficult to stop take a quarter of a teaspoon of cayenne in water, preferably warm, internally, and apply a tourniquet externally.

HICCUPS

As this tends only to be a problem when food is fermenting in the stomach the first rule is to meticulously adhere to the rules of food combining.

I'm sure you have heard about drinking cold water out of the wrong side of a glass. Surprisingly, it often works very effectively, but if it doesn't, take the digestive tincture directly on the tongue, five to seven drops as needed, or encourage the child to sip a cup of fennel tea. Alternatively, encourage her to eat a lemon wedge soaked in angostura bitters. It will certainly get her attention! Breathing into a paper bag, *not a plastic one*, often helps.

INSECT STINGS

First remove the sting by flicking it out with the thumb nail so that the barb comes out cleanly without tearing the skin. If you have an ice-cube available rub it on the area or if not simply suck up and spit out the poisons. Rub tincture of plantain on to the skin or, if you do not have this, chew a plantain leaf into a pulp and apply it as a poultice over the sting or apply a piece of raw onion to it. Administer ten drops of plantain in water every two hours orally until the swelling and itching have subsided.

STINGS IN THE THROAT

For insect stings in the throat, first gargle with four teaspoons of salt in a cup of water and spit the gargle out. The salt water will draw out the poison. Then take ten drops of plantain in water every ten minutes orally and apply a cabbage leaf poultice externally to the neck.

INSECT REPELLENTS

To repel insects eat plenty of garlic or nutritional yeast.

Dr Christopher's Insect Repellent

Combine equal parts of rosemary, basil, wormwood and rue. Crush them together well in a pestle and mortar and pour over olive oil (preferably organic) in proportions of one part of herbs to five parts of oil. Add a dessert spoon of apple cider vinegar and cover the bowl setting it over a radiator for a week. Strain well while the moisture is warm. Measure out the oil and repeat in proportions one part of fresh herbs added to five parts of the oil. Do this two more times and on the third time let the mixture sit over the radiator for at least a couple of weeks. Strain well. You will now have an extremely effective concentrated oil which will keep insects away and is good for the skin at the same time. A little of it dabbed on to the insect sting quickly helps the swelling and itching go away.

To my mind this is far preferable to citronella oil used in natural commercially marketed preparations. Citronella to me smells so nasty it acts as a human repellent not just an insect one!

ITCHING
Poisonous Plants

If the skin has been stung by a poisonous plant but there is no blistering hold the area under running hot water at 49°C (120°F) for a minute or so and then apply tincture of plantain.

RECTAL ITCHING

If it is not the result of bowel or rectal disease or antibiotics, it can sometimes be the result of a poor reaction to coffee, tea, cold drinks, beer, chocolate or foods containing sugar or tomatoes. Take alternate hot and cold sitz baths and apply tincture of golden seal directly to the anal area. Alternatively, try garlic oil applied directly. (See page 150 and check for parasitic infection).

LICE

Lice don't generally hang around a body that is clean and healthy so good personal hygiene and an excellent diet will help to prevent them. If you do have to treat your child use the following formulation which is Dr Christopher's.

Infuse:
6 parts hyssop   *half a part cloves powdered*
1 parts walnut leaves or inner bark   *half a part lobelia powdered*
half a part cinnamon powdered   *half a part of ginger powdered.*

• Strain.

For a child over twelve offer half a cup internally three times a day. For children under the age of twelve, reduce the dosage proportionately a child of six to have a quarter of a cup, for example. Meanwhile bathe the head or body parts affected with black walnut tincture dabbed directly onto the skin.

NIGHTMARES

Make sure your child eats only lightly before retiring and ensure her bowels are working well. Offer her a cup of infused catnip tea before bed and individually select a Bach Flower Remedy to go into it. Try, as far as you can, to be selective about her daily mental input including what she reads and what she sees, and who she talks to because it all adds up.

POISONING

Above all keep the patient calm. Panic merely accelerates the speed with which the poison invades the system. *Seek immediate medical help.* Should the victim have swallowed a poisonous substance some hours before do not waste time by inducing vomiting, get to the hospital quickly. If you don't know what the victim has swallowed and they are unable to tell you or are unconscious describe if possible the container and give all the information you can to the hospital over the phone. They will advise you what is to be done immediately while you wait for an ambulance.

Caustic poisoning

If the substance is caustic **do not** induce vomiting as it will only burn the throat further. Plenty of milk or soya milk will slow its absorption. If you can see the victim is getting drowsy give strong coffee and keep them walking. If the victim is unconscious do not administer anything orally at all. Paracetamol does not induce a coma initially but in large quantities it can damage the liver often fatally so act quickly and get the victim to the hospital with the utmost speed.

Food Poisoning

Follow the treatment recommended for diarrhoea; the colon may be cleared by inducing vomiting with a teaspoon of mustard powder in water. Sooth the aching stomach afterwards with sips of very hot peppermint tea. Combat dehydration with plenty of fluids and chew as many charcoal tablets as possible. Ideally you should give twice the amount of charcoal as the suspected weight of the poison ingested. Powdered Charcoal, stirred into juice, if you can get it, is wonderful for absorbing any kind of toxic material in the gastro-intestinal tract.

RINGWORM

This is a fungoid parasite which needs to be sealed off from the air so paint the area with undiluted lemon juice to form a glaze and continue to do this every few hours until the ringworm is destroyed. Internally administer black walnut tincture according to age and include as much fresh garlic in the diet as possible. Both are excellent anti-fungal treatments.

SHOCK

I find Dr Bach's Rescue Remedy a supreme solution for this. The mother tincture should be diluted four drops in two fluid ounces (50 ml) of pure spring water to which you can add a little brandy as a preservative or, if you don't want to give your child alcohol, cider vinegar. Give four drops of this in a teaspoon (5 ml) of water and hold it on the tongue for thirty seconds before swallowing. Repeat this at least four and up to six times daily. If the patient is unconscious, rub it into the lips or on the wrists (for suppliers see Resources Directory). Alternatively, take one teaspoon of cayenne tincture in hot water or thirty drops of cayenne pepper in a little water. Continue to do this until normal colour returns and if necessary get medical help as quickly as possible. My strong feeling is that the emotional effects of shock need to be helped immediately. Neglected they can reverberate through the system for years causing an insidious build up of all sorts of psychological and physiological problems.

SPRAINS

If you have any doubt at all and think the joint may be fractured seek medical help and in the meanwhile apply an ice pack to the area immediately. I have been known to use a packet of frozen peas in emergencies. If you need an ice pack on an awkwardly shaped area soak a towel in cold water, wring it out until it stops dripping and place it folded on foil in the freezer. Turn the freezer up to maximum. Leave it in there until crystals form but the towel is not frozen solid. When used it will contour itself nicely to the injured area. I here found that if you need to massage an area with ice on a regular basis a good method is to fill a polystyrene plastic cup with water and then freeze. Once frozen peel the cup to below ice level which will then give you a manageable block of ice and a cold resistant handle. Keep the ice moving to avoid skin damage and stop the treatment the moment the skin becomes numb. This type of massage has been found to be very useful in 80 per cent of patients complaining of chronic pain of various types ranging from lower back pain, rheumatoid and osteo arthritis and cancer. Yes children do get arthritis. My youngest patient was six years old. It will supply relief for up to three hours.

As soon as the ice pack is in place elevate the joint to stop effusion. If the fingers and toes turn blue you have overdone it. Once the swelling has reduced somewhat apply a compress of comfrey securing it with a thin elasticated bandage and leave this on for a day. Discourage the patient from moving if at all possible. Do not walk on a sprained ankle. Use crutches if necessary. Enforce complete bed rest for back sprains and apply a sling to immobilise the sprain for a shoulder. Once the swelling has subsided if bruising is present apply arnica tincture frequently.

STIFF NECK

Give warm drinks of sage tea with plenty of honey and lemon in it, dosage according to age. Apply a castor oil poultice to the neck as hot as possible and renew every four hours. Alternatively, massage into the neck deep heat oil (see Resources Directory) or tiger balm and cover it with a warm cloth.

TRAVEL SICKNESS

Simply chewing a piece of fresh ginger root or taking some powdered ginger has proved to be twice as effective for travel sickness as Dramamine.

Now I am prone to almost every type of travel sickness there is and I have found an acupressure point called Nei-Kuan helps relieve all sorts of sickness. It can be found on the surface of the inside of both forearms three finger widths away from the crease of the wrist and in the centre between the two flex tendons. Press this point with the tip of the thumb firmly (obviously short finger nails help here) and repeat as often as necessary. A specially designed wrist strap with a rounded plastic button that will do this for you is available in chemists.

I have found that it also helps to focus on distant objects while travelling in a car or on a train, rather than on nearby ones moving fast. My favourite seat on a plane is over the wheels rather than in the tail which moves more than the rest of the aircraft. On a ship I try to stay on deck as much as I can, no matter what the weather. Gusts of fresh air and sea spray keep my mind focused on better things!

All these pieces of advice may be pertinent for your child.

WARTS

These are a viral infection and should be treated internally as well as externally. Externally paint the area around the wart with olive oil then apply a slice of garlic slightly bruised over the wart, securing with elastoplast. Renew this every day after the child has bathed. Internally give echinacea, the maximum dose for a twelve year-old, being 180 drops of the tincture daily for a week and adjust the dose for smaller children appropriately. Then reduce the dose to ten drops three times a day according to age. Echinacea is an excellent anti-viral tincture.

APPENDIX 1

Some ante-natal tests routinely employed by the medical profession are not only unhelpful they can be harmful.

• URINE TESTING •

A little sugar can often be traced in the urine during pregnancy and unless you are a diabetic may simply mean that you have eaten something sweet recently.

• ROUTINE WEIGH •

One of the first things that will be requested of you is not to gain too much weight. This is because doctors feel that if you do so you may get pre-eclampsia; but the cause of pre-eclampsia is not putting on lots of weight in short periods of time towards the end of a pregnancy but malnutrition. Tom Brewer, a New York physician, who, together with his wife Gail, founded the Society for the Protection of the Unborn through Nutrition (SPUN – see Resources Directory), and who have studied pre-eclampsia extensively, pinpointed nutritional deficiencies as its prime cause. Also known as toxemia, evidenced by elevated blood pressure, protein in the urine, oedema or a rapid weight gain, Brewer has maintained since the 1960s that these physical signs are an indication of ill health or a nutritional deficiency which can lead to problems. Doctors try to correct toxemia with diuretic drugs, restricted salt diets and calorie intake and Brewer maintains that metabolic toxemia of late pregnancy is actually an iatrogenic (physician induced) disease. Brewer suggests intelligent nutritional counselling for all pregnant women as well as rigorous training of doctors in nutrition and emphasis on instructing them to employ scrupulous careful diagnostic procedures in order to distinguish MTLP from conditions which are either normal in pregnancy, such as oedema, or may be indications of other disorders like urinary tract infections or high blood pressure due to too much stress. But doctors continue to confuse these conditions with toxemia.

Weight checks are only really useful if you are incredibly thin or seriously fat. If you are underweight to begin with its actually OK to gain as much as 40 to 50 lbs (18 to 22 kg) without it being an excessive burden to your system. Indeed women who put on only very small amounts of weight during their pregnancies are known to have a higher risk of premature births, abruptio placenta, and toxemia. It is women who are seriously underweight before pregnancy who are more liable to develop these problems and the best way to avoid them is to eat high quality nutritious food (see pages 22–65).

Very rarely if a pregnant woman's weight gain stops abruptly for a couple of months and her uterus does not appear to be growing it could be a sign the foetus is dead. But it is essential to remember that weight gain patterns in pregnancy vary considerably. All foetuses grow in spurts and every woman's pattern of weight gain will be individual.

• VAGINAL EXAMINATION •

This ritual is often done routinely any time from the thirty-third week on, once weekly, but vaginal examinations increase the risk of infection and premature rupture of the membranes which may force a woman into a situation where she has to have a caesarean section.

• ULTRASOUND •

This is still highly experimental and it is worth remembering that it took nearly fifty years for the medical profession to acknowledge that X-rays during pregnancy could lead to an increased risk of leukemia and other cancers for foetuses exposed to them later in life. In 1973, of the sixty-five amniotic fluid specimens taken from patients who had been exposed to ultrasound, thirty-five could not be grown on culture media. Put another way this means that 60 per cent of those women who had been given ultrasound during pregnancy suffered changes in their amniotic fluid.

In fact you are more likely to lose your baby if you are subjected to ultrasound during the course of your pregnancy. Toddlers who have been exposed to ultrasound while in the womb can also suffer from delayed speech and a higher incidence of dyslexia. Unsurprisingly ultrasound has also been found to damage various processes in a pregnant woman's body including her erythrocytes (mature red blood cells) and chorionic gonadatropin levels.

Like all technology the results are only as good as the interpretation and ultrasound as a method of determining gestation is far from accurate. A better way to determine a baby's due date is by feeling the size of the growing uterus and a more accurate way of diagnosing the baby's weight is by determining fundal height. Ultimately the baby will be born when it is ready. The only instance in which ultrasound may be useful is to assist in confirming suspicions of placenta previa (a complication where the placenta is attached close to or at the bottom of the uterus), or to find out exactly how twins are positioned. Usually indicated by a bloody show just before a woman goes into labour, the bleeding occurs when the cervix dilates pulling the placenta away from the lower part of the stretched uterine wall. The bleeding can often be quite heavy and you will be advised to stay in bed until it stops and the danger of the placenta completely detaching has passed. If, during labour, the baby's heartbeat is within the normal range and you are not losing too much blood, a doctor will decide whether the baby can be born safely vaginally. There are very rare cases in which the placenta covers all or most of the cervix and will pull away from the uterine wall completely before the baby is born so that the mother could haemorrhage and the baby would have no oxygen supply at all. This is one of the few justifiable uses of caesarean delivery and almost always the mother and baby emerge from the experience perfectly well.

A final thought; Dr Robert Mendelsohn wrote, 'Ultrasound produces at least two biological effects – heat and a process called "cavitation" in which bubbles are created that expand and contract in response to sound waves. The first time I saw this cavitation process in action, a chiropractor turned on the therapeutic ultra-sound machine in his office and placed a few drops of water on the part of the machine that was applied to the patient. I wish every reader could have been with me to watch that water suddenly boil and bubble.'

• AMNIOCENTESIS •

Amniocentesis is usually recommended to detect genetic abnormalities, when a woman has had a child who was previously born with some type of disorder, to treat serious blood incompatibility or to find out if the foetus's lungs are mature enough before a planned caesarean. In many instances the chance that the procedure itself will cause harm to the foetus is actually greater than the possibility that the foetus has an abnormality. The risks of miscarriage are estimated to be 1.5 per 100 pregnancies and these are mainly the result of the tragic consequences when a needle pokes an eye or injures a vital organ such as a long or major blood vessel of the foetus or RH sensitisation occurs because the mother and baby's blood are mixed. There is also a 3 per cent increase of neo-natal respiratory upset and approximately the same percentage of congenital dislocations of the hip and club feet. My feeling is that any woman over thirty-five who is carrying a much loved and wanted baby should seriously consider these statistics before consenting to this test. Early amniocentesis is now recognised as being so dangerous that in Holland doctors refuse to use it considering it unethical. Robert Mendelsohn has come up with some very interesting research which suggests that Down's Syndrome, far from being the result of tired eggs, is actually caused by the amount of accumulated exposure to X-rays and has nothing to do with one's age. His prophetic views have since been confirmed by studies linked to the aftermath of the Chernobyl disaster, in which nine months after the nuclear accident, Down's Syndrome babies increased six-fold. This rather puts into doubt the alpha foetal protein tests, even supposing they are accurate which they often aren't. The AFP test 'misses about 40 per cent of spina bifida cases, 10 per cent of the anencephaly cases.' It also misses 80 per cent of foetuses with Down's Syndrome.

• THE TRIPLE TEST •

This test is designed to detect Down's Syndrome. In women over thirty-five who are especially worried about this it is worth noting it is only 50 per cent accurate and if you do receive a incorrect positive result you will then be asked to undergo amniocentesis with all the adherent risks of miscarriage.

• CHORIONIC VILLUS SAMPLING (CVS) •

The bad news is you are even more likely to lose your baby with this kind of intervention than with amniocentesis, nor is it accurate. The chances of a false positive result are one in six. The CVS test also carries with it a fairly high risk of the baby being born with limb abnormalities (1 in 200 compared with the normal risk of 1 in 3,100) and in one study that I found really shocking, *all* mothers given CVS, totalling 75, produced a baby with some type of birth defect. The risk of miscarrying as a result of this test is 5 per cent and because it is acknowledged as being fairly inaccurate you will be asked to follow up with an amniocentesis test which will almost double that risk again.

• THE OXYTOXIN CHALLENGE TEST (SOMETIMES CALLED THE CONTRACTION STRESS TEST) •

A woman who has high blood pressure who is running past her due date can sometimes be subjected to this. She is attached to a foetal heart monitor and injected with an oxytoxin-like drug. The foetal heartbeat is monitored during this artificially induced stress and if it plummets significantly during a contraction and stays down it is deemed a natural labour will be too stressful for the foetus or that the foetus could even die before labour begins. In reality just because a woman has a positive oxytoxin challenge test doesn't mean that she or her baby will have difficulty as again, like every other test so far cited, it is far from accurate. Studies indicate that women whose foetuses have slowed heart rates during the OCT have a higher incidence of problems during labour, more still births, smaller babies and unsurprisingly their babies tend to take longer to breathe and move immediately after birth. Common sense suggests to me that some of these problems could be caused by the OCT test itself. A far more accurate, simple and non-interventionist test is the non-stress test.

• NON STRESS TEST •

1. This should only be done towards the end of pregnancy when the foetus is more mature.
2. It is useful when the foetus is overdue.
3. It utilises the observation that the occurrence of accelerations of the foetal heart rate in response to foetal movement or a uterine contraction is a reliable indicator of immediate foetal wellbeing.

4. With a stethoscope or fetoscope the foetal heart rate is listened to for several minutes and recorded for each 15 seconds. If there is any foetal movement during the counting the person carrying out the test needs to put a star or mark next to that 15 second count. Best to have the mother wave her hand whenever she feels movement, although you will probably be able to hear the foetus move yourself.
5. When the time is completed multiply each 15 second number by four in order to get the rate per minute.
6. Normal foetal heart rate should be within normal range of 120 to 160 beats per minute.
7. There is a normal variability of 5 to 15 beats per minute. There may be more with foetal movement.
8. It is good to have acceleration of heartbeat associated with foetal movement.

Another indication that all is well with the foetus is simply to feel regular movement. If the foetus moves at least ten times in a twelve-hour period and at least once in each six-hour period, this is a pretty sure indication that it is not distressed. You can keep a log and record of how many times you feel the foetus move each day and although it will move less vigorously once the head moves down into the pelvis, it will still continue to move when it is awake. This is a much safer non-invasive check on foetal wellbeing than OCT.

Medical Intervention and its Alternatives	
Intervention	**Alternative**
Ultrasound: to diagnose pregnancy	Standard pregnancy test using blood urine together with examination by a skilled doctor
Ultrasound: to determine foetal position	A pregnant woman can be taught to feel the position of the foetus plus examination by a skilled doctor
Ultrasound: to determine foetal heartbeat	Skilled doctor uses a stethoscope
Amniocentesis: to decide on foetal lung maturity	Patience until the woman goes into labour as an indication that it is time for the baby to be born
amniocentesis: to determine genetic defects	None
Oxytoxin Challenge Test	Non-stress testing, keeping regular notes of foetal movements, testing foetal heartbeat during and after vigorous exercise
Diuretics, calorie reduction and sodium-restricted diet for toxemia	Adequate protein in the diet, particularly in the last trimester, a healthy wholefood diet, unrestricted weight gain, plus sodium taken from natural sources in its natural form as found in fruits and vegetables.

• VACCINATIONS •

Most doctors ardently believe that vaccines have successfully wiped out the worst infectious diseases of the last century. Such fervency has inspired them to produce ever more vaccines. American children now receive a total of sixteen vaccinations and multiple booster shots before the age of five, most of these in the first few months of life; and Britain, where the tuberculosis vaccine is administered later, runs roughly parallel.

The problem is no one, as yet, has stopped to examine the possible long-term effect of assaulting an immature immune system with as many as nine different antigens. Dr J. Anthony Morris, once a director of Virology at the Food and Drug Administration and the National Institute of Health is concerned that there is an entire spectrum of reactions somewhere between fever and death which never get reported. These include subtle damage like asthma, learning disabilities, hyper-activity and severe lingering earache. The main problem is not that vaccines don't work, but that they work haphazardly. The theory behind vaccinations assumes that injecting a child with a weakened live or killed virus will force the body to develop antibodies to the disease in the same way as it does when a disease is contracted naturally. The scientific studies so far conducted show that there are a number of vaccines which are capable of raising antibodies to a specific infectious disease in ways which can be measured, **but only for a short period of time**. Even if vaccines are capable of raising antibodies indefinitely this may still have nothing to do with protecting a child from contracting the disease over the long or even the short term. For example large numbers of people who have had illnesses like diphtheria are found never to produce antibodies to the disease. Measles antibodies have been found in the blood of only one in seven vaccinated children who had then gone on to develop measles. In other words they hadn't developed antibodies from either the vaccine or the disease itself. In 1995 the Public Health Laboratory in London found that a quarter of all blood donors between the ages of twenty and twenty-nine had insufficient immunity to diphtheria even though nearly all of them had been vaccinated as babies and this percentage doubled in the fifty to fifty-nine year old age group.

As yet there is no convincing scientific evidence that mass inoculations can take the credit for eliminating any childhood disease. For example diseases like polio operate cyclically. The big polio epidemics of this century were in the first decade and then the 1930s and 1950s. After this period it sharply dropped off to nearly zero. But at the height of the fifties epidemic, after the Salk vaccine was introduced, the vaccine stole the credit instead of nature. Indeed, far from science having anything to do with finally eliminating polio or TB it seems that both diseases took a back seat some years ago and are now beginning to make a comeback – TB in many western countries and polio in parts of Canada. Diphtheria is now rife in Russia and the East. The massive 80 per cent decline in deaths from whooping cough occurred *before* the vaccine was introduced.

Parents are often bullied or frightened into vaccinating their children because they are told that childhood diseases can be a killer, but if a child's immune system is kept running high through good nutrition this is extremely unlikely. Most of the eighty-nine deaths at the height of a measles epidemic in 1990 in America where 27,000 cases were reported were among children of low-income families where poor nutrition predominated, as did failure to treat complications. In the Third World countries where children are markedly vitamin A-deficient measles certainly can kill but there are many studies that have proved that those given vitamin A supplementation are overwhelmingly likely to survive. During the whooping cough epidemic of 1978–9, in low risk areas including Glamorgan, Glasgow and Surrey (all areas where there would be adequate nutrition), there were no cases of permanent brain damage or death among any children, even babies who were considered most at risk. As far as polio is concerned current statistics estimate that only 10 per cent of people exposed to it will actually contract it, and only 1 per cent of those will come down with a parasitic variety, which pans out at 0.01 per cent of those exposed to polio overall and even this tiny percentage may be the result of a special anatomical susceptibility.

Besides all this vaccinations may not actually work at all. In America where at least four different strains from the measles vaccine have been employed, there have been significant numbers of vaccinated children who have nevertheless contracted the disease. In 1986 there was an outbreak of measles in Corpus Christi, Texas, where 99 per cent of the children had already been vaccinated.

Nor has the rubella vaccine, which is usually included in the MMR triple vaccine, performed much better. For a start viruses are notoriously easy to mutate so a vaccine may protect you against only one strain and not another. Ten per cent of girls injected with the rubella vaccine in Italy were shown to be infected by a wild strain of the virus within a few years of receiving their injection.

There are also significant risks associated with every immunisation which comes attached to numerous contra indications. Most of the short-term hazards are known (although rarely explained) but no one as yet knows the long term consequences of injecting foreign proteins into the body of a vulnerable child and so far very little effort as been made to find out. The largest and most definitive study of vaccines was conducted by the Centre for Disease Control and Prevention. It concluded that any child's risk of seizure *triples* within days of receiving either the MMR or DPT vaccines. Seizures, which include epilepsy, convulsions and fainting are already up there as one of the most common conditions in childhood. It affects one in twenty children and these new findings increase that risk to nearly four in twenty. The findings of the CDC were endorsed by the Public Heath Laboratories Service which concluded that the MMR vaccine increased seizure risk five times while the DPT one caused a four-fold increase. The authorities concerned are not agreed as to whether the seizures were caused by individual vaccines or whether the antigen conglomerate of so many simultaneously administered vaccines is causing a general immune system collapse.

Nor should you run away with the misguided belief that vaccines are adequately tested before being injected into vulnerable children. For example the pertussis drug has remained unchanged since its creation in 1912. The bacteria is grown in large stewing pots. Killed with heat and then preserved with formaldehyde which in itself is carcinogenic. Being a whole-cell vaccine means it contains endotoxins and cell-wall substances which were acknowledged to be extremely toxic causing fever, growth interference and death in laboratory animals. To add insult to injury, nowadays a metal salt often made from aluminium is added to heighten the effect of the drug and a further preservative which is a mercury derivative is added. Aluminium and mercury, as you know, are highly toxic to humans.

Some Governments are waking up to the damage that vaccines do. For example in Sweden, Japan and Germany the whooping cough vaccine is now suspended. It has been linked to juvenile diabetes, learning disabilities, infantile spasms, attention deficit disorder and sudden infant death syndrome.

A seemingly simple tetanus vaccine is just as dangerous. The American Sub-committee on Investigations and General Oversight acknowledged that this vaccine can cause high fever, pain, nerve damage to the inner ear, degeneration of the nervous system and anaphylactic shock. The subsequent boosters can cause T-Lymphocyte counts to dive to levels that AIDS victims are normally saddled with. Unhappily some Governments, including our own, are slow learners. New Zealand got there the hard way. It was one of the first countries to adopt a universal programme of compulsory vaccination of hepatitis B for all new-born babies in 1988. After only three months of the programme the contra-indications began to be reported and then continued flooding in for a year. They included lethargy, malaise, diarrhoea, asthma, arthritis, Guillain-Barre syndrome, faintness, pallor, loss of consciousness and worrying drops in blood pressure. One in fifty children suffered one or more of these effects after their first dose and a number of children also suffered from post-natal jaundice for two to three weeks after immunisation. By 1992 the chastened New Zealand Health Department bought the vaccination programme to an abrupt halt.

Vaccinations bring with them their own new or mutated diseases. For example it has been estimated that 3 per cent of babies born to mothers given hepatitis B vaccine then go on to develop a mutant of HBV. There is also a worrying connection between the growing prevalence of penicillin resistant pneumococcal meningitis and HIB vaccination. Provocation polio after a just-in-case injection has long been recognised and accepted as a fact in Britain and America. Indeed multiple injections may be responsible for 25 per cent of cases of paralysis during epidemics of polio making children 25 per cent more susceptible to the disease during non-epidemic periods. The measles and tuberculosis vaccines have been linked with the current epidemic of myalgic encephalomyelitis, sometimes called chronic fatigue syndrome, particularly among children. There is evidence that suggests that the symptoms of ME are partly the result of a dysfunction in the body caused by an antibody response to incomplete, dead or even latent viruses such as those in the weakened version of vaccine viruses. Michel Odent discovered that those children immunised against whooping cough were six times more likely to have asthma as those who weren't.

• NATURAL SOLUTIONS •

1. Breast feed your child if at all possible from the day of birth for as long as possible and for at least six months (see pages 123–125).
2. Boost your child's immunity by giving them a varied wholefood diet and ensure that it is rich in natural beta carotene. The *Lancet* has reported that giving vitamin A to children with severe measles, for example. lessens the complications or chances of dying. Children with marginal liver stores of vitamin A may develop an acute vitamin A deficiency resulting in eye damage and the possibility of an increase in deaths from respiratory diseases and diarrhoea.
3. Avoid antibiotics except in cases of acute bacteria middle-ear infection.
4. Avoid operations and particularly ensure, if at all possible, that your child keeps her tonsils intact. As Robert Mendelsohn, noted, 'The tonsils and adenoids are lymphoid tissues, which are the primary site of the body's immunologic activity against disease. Because they are the interceptors of bacteria entering your child's throat, it is inevitable that they become infected, swollen and inflamed. If they are removed, your child's first line of defence against infection has gone and the responsibility is transferred to the lymph nodes in his neck. His body's immunologic competence is reduced and there will be an increased risk that your child will become a victim of Hodgkin's disease.' Chronic infections, particularly of the ear or throat, can be reduced by avoiding dairy products which are often a prime culprit or white refined products and attending to allergies or nutritional deficiencies.

   A child's immune defences start in the mucosa of the mouth and nose which are recipients and buffers for the impact of dangerous microbes on the bloodstream, well before an antibody response is necessary. In cases of natural immunity only small amounts of antigenic material can make their way through this initial line of defence deeper into the child's body and these are just enough to trigger an immune response but not so overwhelming that they engulf the child's natural resistance. This is natural immunity at its best.
5. Remember the healing power of fever (see pages 152–4). Work with it.
6. Work with childhood illnesses on a natural basis (see chapter 9). As Robert Mendelsohn has observed, hospitals are places where people go to get sick so don't allow your child to be admitted to one unless her condition is so serious that her life is in danger. Remember relatively few childhood ailments require hospitalisation but far too many children are hospitalised needlessly simply because it is more convenient for their doctor. Most illnesses and accidental injuries can be treated as effectively in an emergency room, doctor's office or an outpatients clinic with hospitalisation. It is often the case that your child will receive better and safer care at home. Besides this the hazards of hospitalisation for young children and babies are not limited to the physical risks. There may be

damaging psychological and emotional consequences as well. For a child a simple separation from her mother or family for any period of time can be an extremely traumatic experience as well as a frightening one.

Avoid sending your child to nursery or day-care facilities too early. It was Mendelsohn who alerted the world to the problem of warehousing large groups of non-toilet trained babies. Many day-care facilities are suffering an epidemic of HIB caused meningitis.

APPENDIX 2

SUB FERTILITY

It wasn't long ago that the problem that women were most concerned about was preventing fertility but for a growing number of couples now the problem is infertility. About 25 per cent of all couples conceive the first month they try; 50 per cent will have succeeded within six months, and 85 per cent within a year. Of the remaining 15 per cent, one quarter will conceive in the following year.

• MALE INFERTILITY •

In about 40 per cent of these cases the problem is due to the male partner and usually the trouble is one of low sperm count. There have been an increasing number of articles hitting the headlines about the fact that the quality of modern day sperm is being heavily affected by insecticides. Other factors which impair sperm production can be due to heavy metal poisoning, radiation exposure (including X-rays) or prolonged drug use, both of recreational and prescribed drugs, as well as an undetected infection leading to atrophy of the testicles, or a trauma or blow to the testicles. Sometimes a nasty case of adult mumps will effect fertility as of course will kidney failure, chronic lung disease (usually from smoking), thyroid deficiency, calcium, vitamin E or zinc deficiency. A low sperm count has been detected in regular drinkers of alcohol. Obstruction of the seminal tract itself may be congenital or due to inflammation of the prostate, inflammation of the testicles or any other local inflammatory process as well as more wide-spread infections of the kidneys or liver.

With repeated ejaculations the numbers of sperm in the ejaculate decline, so if your partner has ejaculated several times over the preceding few days, conception is less likely to occur on the day you ovulate because his semen will contain insufficient sperm. For this reason it is probably best to abstain from intercourse for two to three days before ovulation is expected to occur.

On a woman's part if she stands up and walks around immediately after making love most of the seminal fluid will leak out of her vagina. To give as many sperm as possible a chance of reaching the fallopian tubes where the egg cells will be, it is a good idea to lie quietly on the bed for at least twenty minutes after making love with your bottom raised up slightly on a pillow and the knees bent in towards the chest. Twenty per cent of those men who are infertile are found to produce high levels of superoxide radicals in their semen and vitamin E which acts as an antioxidant, will mop up their superoxide radicals. Infertile men should realise that sperm cannot be manufactured in excessive heat. This includes heat from very hot showers, baths, saunas, Turkish baths, as well as tight fitting underwear and trousers or electrical blankets at night. So underwear should be loose, boxer shorts are ideal, and made of cotton. Cold showers as well as cold sitz baths on a twice daily basis are an excellent idea, particularly before intercourse. Smoking decreases the sexual capability of a man by damaging the minute blood vessels that supply blood to the penis so the obvious solution is to stop smoking. Studies in North Carolina in the United States show that drinking four cups of coffee a day and smoking more than twenty cigarettes was a dangerous combination for male fertility. Margarine has also been implicated in low sperm counts. Sperm of an inappropriate consistency can be corrected by large doses of vitamin C. The classic herbs for correcting male infertility are gotu kola, damiana, and saw palmetto. To any formulation I use I normally also like to add prickly ash and a touch of cayenne pepper to assist the circulation.

• FEMALE INFERTILITY •

A very common cause of female infertility is blocked or partly blocked fallopian tubes which can be the result of previously undetected pelvic infections particularly chlamydia. Some women develop antibodies to their partners sperm as part of an allergic reaction. This can be corrected by having your partner use a condom for a month during which time your own antibodies will decrease. Other causes in infertility include a lack of periods, tension, stress and tiredness, cervical polyps, inflammation of the cervix or ovaries, fibroids, cystic ovaries, endometriosis and, more interestingly, a lack of orgasm during intercourse. The strong muscular contractions a female orgasm produces helps to push sperm from the uterus into the fallopian tubes where eggs are fertilised and aided by such an orgasm sperm can travel this distance in a mere fifteen minutes, fifty times faster than it would take if they swam without help. While male impotence has always been an obvious factor in infertility until recent studies at the Hammersmith hospital in London, female impotence, or the inability to achieve an orgasm, has never until now been on the agenda. When infertility in a woman is described as idiopathic, meaning no one knows the cause for certain, this aspect of infertility might well be worth considering.

It has been proved that the pill and STDs affect fertility as does vitamin E deficiency, diabetes and steroids. Apparently, women whose mothers smoked when they were pregnant are only 50 per cent as fertile as women who were not exposed in this way in utero and when working with infertile couples I always check the possibility of heavy metal intoxication as well as B_{12} and iron deficiencies.

• OVULATION TIMING SELF-TEST •

It is as well to check if you are under thirty and have been trying to conceive for more than six months without success that you are not consistently making love on infertile days of the month and you can do this by using a temperature chart detecting the change in your cervical mucus, or using a chemically impregnated dipstick to detect the LH in your urine samples (for availability see Resources Directory). While your natural fertility tends to decline after the age of thirty, if you are a woman who has had a child or a previous pregnancy and are unable to conceive both of you are advised to have a complete diagnostic evaluation. The diagnostic tests that specialists use may include using tubes, needles or viewing instruments, radiation, anaesthetics and dye materials, none of which I would recommend and all of which are capable of making the problem worse rather than better.

• INFERTILITY DRUGS •

Nor do I feel at all happy about the infertility drugs that are issued. Clomid, for example, causes flushes in 10 per cent of the women who use it and ovarian enlargement in 14 per cent. Other side effects include blurred vision, double vision, spots in front of the eyes, after images, sensitiveness to artificial light, floaters, waves, cataracts, detachment of the posterior vitreous, spasming of the blood vessels, thrombosis of the retinal arteries, abdominal distention, pelvic pain, nausea and vomiting, increased appetite, constipation, diarrhoea, breast discomfort, abnormal menstrual bleeding, dryness of the vagina, headaches, dizziness, light-headedness, vertigo, nervous tension, insomnia and fatigue, depression, increased urinary frequency and skin rashes, hair loss, hair dryness, weight gain or weight loss, jaundice and fluid in the abdomen. As Eli Lilley once pertinently remarked, no drug is worth its salt without side effects, but this seems to me way too high a price to pay.

If you are already pregnant when you take Clomid it has been known to jeopardise the health of the baby in utero including the potential for congenital heart disease, Down's syndrome, club foot, congenital intestinal conditions, abnormal position of the urethra or opening, a small head, harelip, cleft palate, congenital hip displacement, birthmarks, undescended testicles, extra fingers, conjoined twins, inguinal hernia, umbilical hernia, fused fingers, funnel chest, muscle disorders, dermoid cysts, spina bifida and other defects. All this on top of the potential of multiple births. All other fertility drugs contain risks both to the baby and yourself on about the same level as these. Robert Mendelsohn advises staying away from fertility drugs for very good reasons. Remember you always have the choice and my first option would be to try the natural way first before getting involved in the more problematical chemical alternatives.

• HOLISTIC TREATMENT •

From my own experience I've found that too many infertile couples think only of their reproductive organs when the problem is likely to be far more wide ranging. I have had a huge amount of success in this area by using a holistic approach. I begin with the supposition that nature cannot sprout healthy seed in unhealthy soil so treatment normally includes systematic detoxification. Which systems need detoxifying is determined by an iridology test. In both sexes an inadequate flow of energy circulating through the reproductive organs will depress fertility and this is often due to imbalances in hormones caused by poor diet and a stressful life style. The treatment I use may sound radical to some but I have a very high rate of success and a wall covered in pictures of babies which doctors and specialists pronounced were impossible, a source of deep joy and satisfaction to me.

Systemic detoxification is discussed in many of my previous books including the *Holistic Woman's Herbal* listed in the bibliography. It includes short vegetable juice fasts of five consecutive days every fortnight with a vegan diet in between including plenty of raw and sprouted foods. Sometimes I insist that this diet remains totally raw and organic for the first month or two and while systemic detoxification is going on I suggest barrier contraception is used to stop the possibility of any conception until the soil is ripe. Obviously I remove alcohol, tea, coffee, sugar and salt from the diet altogether, encourage the use of as much organic produce as possible, particularly presoaked and low heated grains and sprouted grains and beans and seeds and all water has to be filtered. I will often use specific superfoods like spirulina, chlorella, beetroot powder, purple dulse, the inner peels from oranges and lemons, rose hips, etc., depending on the outcome of the vega or iridology test. I nearly always begin by cleaning out the bowel of both partners and then I will suggest endocrine balances which are particularly useful in the case of hormone imbalance including motherwort, agnus castus, false unicorn, dong quai, red raspberry, squawvine, blessed thistle, wild yam and fennel. I make a good female fertility tonic which includes equal parts of damiana, wild yam, liquorice, Siberian ginseng, oat seed, gota kola, ginger, false unicorn, agnus castus and motherwort. The herbs are finely powdered and mixed together and the dose is two capsules three times a day with meals.

Dianne Bjarnson has told me of George Wooton, an MD practising in Hurley, New York, who runs a programme that is even more radical than mine and claims close to 100 per cent success rate. His programme consists of a five day fast on nothing but purified water together with rigorous bowel cleansing beginning from the third day and subsequently three more weeks of raw fruits and vegetables only. He suggests that on this programme alone nearly all of the people he has treated are pregnant within three to four months.

RESOURCES DIRECTORY

_____

• PRENATAL CARE •

Foresight (The Association for Promotion of Pre-conceptual Care).
Mrs P Barnes, The Old Vicarage, Church Lane, Witley, Godalming, Surrey GU5 5PN
Tel: 01483 427839 (Stamped addressed envelope for 29p appreciated.)

• MERCURY-FREE DENTISTRY •

Jack Levenson,
  1 Welbeck House,
  62 Welbeck Street,
  London
  W1N 7SB
  Tel: 0171 486 3127 (Stamped addressed envelope appreciated.)

Hesham El-Essawy,
  121 Harley Street,
  London
  W1N 1DH
  Tel: 0171 935 3960

• MERCURY TESTING •

John Morley,
  140 Harley Street,
  London
  W1N 1AH
  Tel: 0171 487 2617

• SUPPLIERS •

Holistic Research Company
Brighthaven,
Robin's Lane,
Lolworth,
Cambridge
CB3 8HH
Tel: 01954 781074

This company supplies wheat grass juice presses as well as good juicers. Also the supplier of enema kits.

Cytoplan
205 West Malvern Road,
West Malvern,
Worcestershire
UR14 4BB
Tel: 01684 577777
Suppliers of enema kits.

GB Nursery Products Limited
13 Pollards Hill West,
Norbury,
London
SW16 4NV
Tel: 0181 764 7936

This company supplies what can best be described as a life saver as far as crying babies are concerned and in my time I have given many away as a welcome-to-the-world gift to mothers and their new babies, all of whom have said it works excellently. It is a string bag which is suspended from a hook in the ceiling in which a baby basket can be placed. It is called a lullaby. It will rock the baby to sleep automatically and can be used in any doorway or ceiling in the house.

Comfort and Joy
Baytree Cottage,
Eastleach,
Nr Cirencester,
Gloucestershire
GL7 3NL
Tel: 0136 7850278
This company supplies mother and baby skin care products of high standard.

BioCare Limited
54 Northfield Road,
Kings Norton,
Birmingham
B30 1JH
Tel: 0121 433 3727

BioCare's products are available direct from the company through herbal practitioners. They make a particularly excellent range of probiotics including ones suitable for babies and toddlers as well as Cervagyn cream to treat candida vaginally.

Bioforce UK Limited
Olympic Business Park,
Dundonald,
Ayrshire
KA2 9BE
Tel: 01563 851177

I have dealt with this company now for many years and greatly admire the fact that by and large they are unique among herbal manufacturers for using only freshly harvested herbs in their tinctures. The herbs are cultivated in a remote north-eastern corner of Switzerland between 800 to 1500 feet above sea level which encourages the condensation of the healing properties in them. In other words they have to be hardy and powerful to survive at this height. This company is also particularly strict about harvesting according to strict protocols. For example, echinacea purpurea is harvested when it reaches three to four feet in height when fifty per cent of the flowers are in bloom and fifty per cent in bud. Harvesting takes place after midday. While many professional herbalists in practice, including myself, are particularly keen to harvest their own herbs freshly whenever possible, most commercially available herbal tinctures are not manufactured to Bioforce's particularly high standards. All Bioforce's products are readily available in health food shops including Diabetisan for the treatment of hypoglycaemia and iron water for anaemia, veleriacom sleeping tablets and valeriana zincum for depression.

The Herbal Apothecary
103 The High Street,
Syston,
Leicester
LE7 1GQ
Tel: 01162 2602690

Are also suppliers of powdered herbs and gelatine and vegetarian gelatine capsules. Please note: before ordering capsules specify if you require vegetarian ones and minimum order is 500. Herbs cannot be supplied in less than half a kilo at a time. Various excellent herbal creams suitable for babies are also available and are made from natural ingredients strictly free of synthetics.

A Nelson & Company Limited,
  5 Endeavour Way,
  Wimbledon,
  London
  SW19 9UE
  Tel: 0181 946 8527
Makes a superb range of herbal ointments and creams. I particularly like this company because they use, as Bioforce does, as much fresh base herbs as they can. Scientific testing using chromatography proves that fresh herb preparations contain more of the active constituents and are more stable compared to their counterparts manufactured from dried herbs.

Potters
  Leyland Mill Lane,
  Wigan,
  Lancashire
  WN1 2SB
  Tel: 01942 234761
This company makes an excellent range of herbal syrups for coughs and colds (which need to be diluted for babies), as well as herbal tonics. Potters also supply unsulphured molasses to Health Food shops.

Baldwin's
  173 Walworth Road,
  London
  SE17 1RW
  Tel: 0171 703 5550
This company sells small amounts of herbs by post and have a fascinating shop which, if you're ever in London, is well worth a visit.

D. Napier & Sons
  18 Bristo Place,
  Edinburgh,
  Scotland
  EH1 1EZ
  Tel: 0131 225 5542 for herbal consultations and all other queries.
For Mail Order: Napiers Mail Order Limited, Forest Bank, Barr, Ayrshire, KA26 9TN
Tel: 0146 586 1625

Kitty Campion
> The Natural Health & Iridology Centre,
> 25 Curzon Street,
> Basford,
> Newcastle-under-Lyme,
> Staffordshire
> ST5 0OP
> Tel: 01782 711592

Supplier of T-Tree pessaries, skin brushes, douche and enema kits and most other composite herbal formulas including the deep heat oil mentioned in this book and the supplier of the Superfoods discussed on page 00. Kitty Campion also teaches many courses about herbal medicine and vegan cookery.

• SUPERFOODS •

Spirulina & Biogenic Aloe Vera juice is available from:

Xxynergy
> Lower Elsted,
> Midhurst,
> West Sussex
> GU29 0JT
> Tel: 01730 813642

This company imports extremely high-quality spirulina from the clean waters around New Zealand, so I particularly condone the purity and the excellence of their product. They are suppliers of biogenic aloe vera juice which is organically grown and prepared in a unique way which does not denature or destroy its delicate enzymes and vital biogenic stimulators. I know of no comparable aloe vera juice on the market. They also supply aloe vera sprays in pump bottles which do not upset the environment.

Marigold Health Foods Limited
> Unit 10 St Pancras Commercial Centre,
> London
> NW1 0BY
> Tel: 0171 267 7368

This company sells superb nutritional yeast flakes under the brand name Engevita.

Floradix is available in health food shops.

● MANUKA HONEY ●

An organic honey. This amazing naturally healing honey is available from:
The New Zealand Natural Food Company Limited
9 Holt Close,
Highgate Wood,
London
N10 3HQ
Tel: 0181 444 5660

● ASSOCIATIONS ●

Vegan Society
7 Battle Road,
St Leonards on Sea,
East Sussex
TN37 7AA
Tel: 01424 427393
An organisation for Vegans.

Viva
PO Box 212,
Crewe,
Cheshire
CW1 4SD
Tel: 01270 522500
Promotes vegan and vegetarian lifestyles. (Enclose an sae for information)

The European Herbal Association of which Kitty Campion is the treasurer will supply a list of fully qualified herbal practitioners trained by Kitty Campion of the College of Herbs and Natural Healing, or with the National Institute of Herbal Medicine, or the General Council and Register of Consultant Medical Herbalists. Write to:

The Herb Society
134 Buckingham Palace Road,
London
SW1W 9SA
Tel: 0171 823 5583

• CAMPAIGNING •

Hyperactive Children Support Group
59 Meadowside,
Angering,
Littlehampton,
Sussex
BN16 4BW
Tel: 01903 725182
This is a well established mutual self-help group for parents of hyperactive children offering practical support and advice as well as literature and they sponsor research in addition to campaigning effectively on relevant issues alongside other organisations.

National Pure Water Association
17 Sycamore Lane West,
Bretton,
Wakefield,
West Yorkshire
WF4 4JR
Tel: 01924 830097
This is an organisation which sends out regular newsletters and is interested in the quality of water and specifically campaigns against fluoridation of water.

The Soil Association
86–88 Colston Street,
Bristol
BF1 5BB
Tel: 0117 9290661
An organisation that vouchsafes for the safety of organic produce.

Action on Smoking and Health (ASHO)
10 Gloucester Place,
London W1.
Tel: 0171 935 3519
Publishes information leaflets and advice on how to give up

National Childbirth Trust
Alexandra House,
Oldham Terrace,
Acton,
London
W3 6NH.
Tel: 0181 992 8637
An organisation interested in empowering women to have the type of delivery they would like.

National Childbirth Trust
Stockbridge Health Centre,
1 India Place,
Edinburgh
EH3 6EH
Tel: 0131 225 9191

National Childbirth Trust
Orla Hastings,
5 Grange Manor Road,
Rathfarmham,
Dublin 16
Tel: 00 3531 4935969

The Birthing Tub Company
24 Seasaw Way,
Brighton,
Sussex
BN2 5LH
Tel: 01273 885775

Splashdown Water Birth Services
C/o Jane Ingrey,
17 Wellington Terrace,
Harrow on the Hill,
Middlesex
HA1 3EP
Tel: 0181 422 9308

This company will ship pools anywhere in the UK. Together with mail order books, videos, workshops for pregnant couples and organizer of international conferences and EMBE midwife approved study courses.

• GIVING BIRTH •

Caroline Flint Midwifery Services
34 Elm Quay Court,
Nine Elm Lane,
London
SW8 5DE
Tel: 0171 498 2322.

This is a private home birth service offering ante-natal classes and ante-natal care as well as post natal care for four weeks and mother's help for two weeks after birth or alternatively help with arranging an NHS home birth.

The Birth Centre
 37 Caverton Road,
 London
 SW17 0QW
 Tel: 0181 767 8294
A private birth centre adjacent to a high-tech maternity unit.

Society to Support Home Confinement
 Lidgate Lane,
 Wolsingham,
 Bishop Auckland,
 County Durham
 DL13 3HA
 Tel: 09565 528044

The La Leche League of Great Britain
 Box BM3424,
 London
 WC1N 3XX
 Tel: 0171 242 1278
This operates internationally around the world and offers excellent help and support and advice on breast feeding.

Active Birth Centre
 25 Bickerton Road,
 London
 N19 5JT
 Tel: 0171 561 9006

• MIDWIVES •

Independent Midwifes Association
 94 Auckland Road,
 Upper Norwood,
 London
 SE19 2DB

ARM (Association of Radical Midwives),
 62 Greetby Hill,
 Ormskirk,
 Lancashire
 L39 2DT
 Tel: 01695 572776
Stamped addressed envelope appreciated.

• ESSENTIAL OILS •

Daniele Ryman's Essential Oils can be purchased by mail order by writing to her at the Marguerite Maury Clinic, Park Lane Hotel, Piccadilly, London W1.

Butterbur & Sage
  Mercantiles House,
  99–101 St Leonards Road,
  Windsor,
  Berkshire
  SL4 3BZ
  Tel: 01734 314484

I have not encountered essential oils commercially available made to the extremely high standards this company employs, and most experienced aromatherapists tend to agree with me.

• VACCINATION •

Organisations who will supply parents with information include:

The Informed Parent
  29 Grayhound Road,
  Sutton,
  Surrey
  SM1 4BY (Please send an sae)

Dissatisfied Parents Together
  128 Branch Road,
  Vienna,
  Vermont 22180
  USA

The Immunisation Awareness Society of Finland
  Box 217,
  SF-01300,
  Vantaa,
  Finland

What Doctor's Don't Tell You
  4 Wallace Road,
  London
  N1 2PG
  Tel: 0171 354 4592

This company have published some excellent information on vaccination as well as the relatively new publication called *Mothers Know Best.*

The British Anti-vivisectionist Association
   PO Box 82,
   Kingswood,
   Bristol
   BS15 1YF
Also supply some interesting information on vaccinations. (Please enclose an sae.)

• COLONIC IRRIGATION THERAPISTS •

Please contact Kitty Campion for a list of colonic therapists personally trained by herself.

BIBLIOGRAPHY

Campion, Kitty, *Holistic Woman's Herbal*, Bloomsbury, London (1995)

Grant, Helen, Dr., *The Bitter Pill*

Grant, Helen, Dr., *Sexual Chemistry*, Mandarin paperbacks London (1994)

Kelly, John & Verny, Thomas, Dr., *The Secret Life of the Unborn Child*, Sphere Books, London (1982)

Kitzinger, Sheila, *Homebirth*, Dorling and Kindersley, London (1991)

Klaper, MD., Michael, *Pregnancy, Children and the Vegan Diet*, Gentle World inc., Hawaii (1987)

Mendelsohn, MD., Robert, S., *Male Practice (How Doctors Manipulate Women)*, Contemporary Books inc., Chicago (1982)

Odent, Michel, *The Nature of Birth and Breastfeeding*, Bergin and Garvey, Westport, Conneticut, London, (1982)

BOTANICAL INDEX

Aconite, *Aconitum Napellus*
Agrimony, *Agrimonia Enpatoria*
Alfalfa, *Medicago Sativa*
Allspice, *Pimento Officinalis*
Almond, *Amygdalus Communis*
Aloe, *Aloe Vera*
Angelica, *Angelica Archangelica*
Anise, *Pimpinella Anisum*
Aniseed, *Pimpinella Anisum*
Arnica, *Arnica Montana*
Arrowroot, *Maranta Arundinaceae*
Artichoke, *Cynara Scolymus*
Ash, *Fraxinus Excelsior*
Autumn Crocus, *Colchicum Autumnale*

Balm, Lemon, *Melissa Officinalis*
Balm of Gilead, *Populus Gileadensis*
Barley, *Hordeum Distichon*
Basil, *Ocimum Basilicum*
Bay Laurel, *Laurel Nobilis*
Bayberry, *Myrica Cerifera*
Bearberry, *Arctostaphylos Uva-ursi*
Belladonna, *Atropa Belladonna*
Benzoin, *Styrax Benzion*
Bergamot, *Monarda Didyma*
Beth Root, *Trillium Pendulum*
Betony (Wood), *Stachys Betonica*
Bilberry, *Vaccinium Myrtillus*
Birch, *Betula Alba*
Black Cohosh, *Cimicifuga Racemosa*
Black Horehound, *Ballota Nigra*
Black Walnut, *Juglans Nigra*
Blessed Thistle, *Cnicus Benedictus*
Blue Cohosh, *Caulophyllum Thalictroides*
Blue Flag, *Iris Versicolor*

Couch Grass, *Agropyrum Repens*
Cowslip, *Primula Veris*
Cramp Bark, *Viburnum Opulus*
Cranberry, *Vaccinum Macrocarpon*
Cucumber, *Cucumis Sativa*
Cudweed Marsh, *Ghaphalium Uliginosum*
Currant (Red), *Ribes Rubrum*

Daisy, *Bellis Perennis*

Juniper, *Juniperus Communis*

Kava Kava, *Piper Methysticum*
Kelp, *Fucus Vesiculosus*

Lady's Mantle, *Alchemilla Vulgaris*
Lady's Slipper, *Cypripedium Pubescens*
Lavender, *Santolina*
Cotton Lavender, *Chamaecy Parissum*
English Lavender, *Lavandula Vera*
Lemon, *Citrus Limonum*
Lemon Balm, *Melissa Officinalis*
Lettuce, *Lactuca Virosa*
Lily (White Water), *Nymphaea Odorata*
Lime, *Citrus Acida*
Linseed (Flax), *Linum Usitatissimum*
Liquorice, *Glycyrrhiza Glabra*
Lobelia, *Lobelia Inflata*
Loosestrife (Purple), *Lythrum Salicaria*
Lovage, *Levisticum Officinale*
Lungwort, *Sticta Pulmonaria*
Lupin, *Leguminosae*

Malefern, *Dryopteris Feliz-mas*
Mandrake, *Atropa Mandragora*
Marigold, *Calendula Officinalis*
Marjoram:
(Sweet), *Origanum Marjorana*
(Wild), *Origanum Vulgare*
Meadowsweet, *Filipendula Ulmaria*
Mimosa, *Mimosa Fragigolia*
Mint (Spear), *Mentha Viridis*
Mistletoe, *Viscum Album*
Moss (Icelandic), *Cetraria Islandica*
Moss (Irish), *Chondrus Crispus*

Moss (Sphagnum), *Sphagnum Cymbifolium*
Motherwort, *Leonurus Cardiaca*
Mugworth, *Artemisia Vulgaris*
Mullein, *Verbascum Thapsus*
Mustard:
  (Black), *Brassica Nigra*
  (White), *Brassica Alba*
Myrrh, *Commiphora Myrrha*

Nasturtium, *Tropaeolum Majus*
Neroli (Orange), *Citrus Aurantium*
Nettles, *Urticaceae*
Nutmeg, *Myristica Fragrans*

Oak, *Lavercus Robur*
Oats, *Avena Sativa*
Olive, *Olea Europaea*
Onion, *Allium Cepa*
Orange:
  (Bitter), *Citrus Vulgaris*
  (Sweet), *Citrus Aurantium*
Orchard (Wild), *Orchid Masculata*
Oregon Grape Root, *Berberis Aquifolium*
Origanum, *Ulgare Aureum*
Orris Root, *Iris Florentina*

Pansy, *Viola Tricolor*
Parsley, *Petroselinum Sativum*
Passion Flower, *Anemone Pusatilla*
Pan d'arco (Taheebo), *Tabenia Impetiginosa*
Peach, *Prunus Persica*
Pellitory of the Wall, *Parietaria Officinalis*
Penny Royal, *Mentha Pulegium*
Peppermint, *Mentha Piperita*
Periwinkle (Greater), *Vinca Major*
Pilewort, *Ranunculus Ficaria*
Pine, *Pinacaea*
Plaintain, *Plantago Major*
Pleurisy Root, *Asclepias Tuberose*
Poke Root, *Phytolacca Decandra*
Pomegranate, *Punica Granatum*
Poppys:
  (Red), *Papaver Rhoeas*
  (White), *Papaver Somniferium*
Prickly Ash, *Xanthoxylum Americanum*

Primrose, *Primula Vulgaris*
Privet, *Liqustrum Vulgare*
Psyllium, *Plantago Psyllium*
Pulsatilla, *Anemone Pulsatilla*
Purslane:
   (Green), *Portulaca Oleracea*
   (Golden), *Portulaca Sativa*

Quassia (Bark), *Picraena Excelsa*
Quince, *Pyrus Cydonia*

Raspberry, *Rubus Idaeus*
Rest-Harrow, *Ononis Arvensis*
Rhubarb (Turkey), *Rheum Palmatum*
Rose, *Rosecaea*
Rosehip, *Rosa Canina*
Rosemary, *Rosemarinus Officinalis*
Rue, *Ruta Graveolens*

Sage, *Salvia Officinalis*
Sandalwood (Yellow), *Santalum Album*
Sassafras, *Sassafras Officinale*
Savory:
   (Summer), *Satureia Hortensis*
   (Winter), *Satureia Montano*
Saw Palmetto, *Sarenoa Serrulata*
Scabious, *Field Scabiosa Arvensis*
Scullcap (Virquinian), *Scutellaria Lateriflora*
Seaweed (General), *Fucus Vesiculosis*
Self-heal, *Prunella Vulgaris*
Senna, *Cassia Acutifolia*
Shepherd's Purse, *Capsella Bursa-Pastoris*
Skunk Cabbage, *Symplocar Pus Foctidus*
Soap Wort, *Saponaria Officinalis*
Solomon's Seal, *Polygonatum Multiflorum*
Sorrel:
   (French), *Rumex Scatatus*
   (Garden), *Rumex Acetosa*
Southernwood, *Field Artemisia Campestria*
Speedwell, *Common Veronica Officinalis*
Squaw Vine, *Mitchella Repens*
Squill, *Urginea Scilla*
St John's Wort, *Hypericum Perforatum*
Stillingia, *Stillingia Sylvatica*
Stone Root, *Collinsonia Canadensis*

Strawberry, *Frangaria Vesca*
Sumac Smooth, *Rhus Glabia*
Sunflower, *Helianthus Annvus*

Tansy, *Tanacetum Vulgare*
Tea Tree, *Melalenca Alternifolia*
Thuja, *Thuja Occidentalis*
Thyme:
  (Garden), *Thymus Vulgaris*
  (Wild), *Thymus Serpyllum*
Toad Flax, *Linaria Vulgaris*
Tobacco, *Nicotiana Tabacum*
Tormentil, *Potentilla Tormentilla*
Tumeric, *Curcuma Longa*

Unicorn (False), *Chamaelirium Luteum*
Unicorn (True), *Aletris Farinosa*
Uva-Ursi, *Arctostaphylos Uva-Ursi*

Valerian, *Valeriana Officinalis*
Vervain (Blue), *Verbena Officinalis*
Vine (General), *Vitis Vinifera*
Violet (Sweet), *Viola Odorata*

Watercress, *Nasturtium Officinale*
Willow (White), *Salix Alba*
Wild Indigo, *Baptisia Tunctoria*
Willow-Herb (Rosebay), *Epilobium Angustifolium*
Winter Green, *Gaultheria Procumbens*
Witch Hazel, *Hamamelis Virginiana*
Woodruff, *Asperula Odorata*
Wormwood (Common), *Artemisia Absinthium*

Yam (Wild), *Dioscorea Villosa*
Yarrow, *Achillea Millefolium*

INDEX